Educating Students With Autism Spectrum Disorder

A Model for High-Quality Coaching

Educating Students With Autism Spectrum Disorder

A Model for High-Quality Coaching

Joshua K. Harrower, PhD, BCBA-D
Louis G. Denti, PhD
Marcia Weber-Olsen, PhD, CCC-SLP

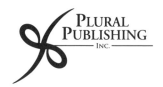

PLURAL
PUBLISHING
INC.

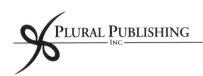

5521 Ruffin Road
San Diego, CA 92123

e-mail: info@pluralpublishing.com
Website: http://www.pluralpublishing.com

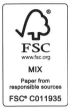

Typeset in 11/14 Garamond by Flanagan's Publishing Services, Inc.
Printed in the United States of America by McNaughton & Gunn, Inc.

For permission to use material from this text, contact us by
Telephone: (866) 758-7251
Fax: (888) 758-7255
e-mail: permissions@pluralpublishing.com

Every attempt has been made to contact the copyright holders for material originally printed in another source. If any have been inadvertently overlooked, the publishers will gladly make the necessary arrangements at the first opportunity.

Library of Congress Cataloging-in-Publication Data

Harrower, Joshua K., author.
   Educating students with autism spectrum disorder : a model for high-quality coaching / Joshua K. Harrower, Louis G. Denti, Marcia Weber-Olsen.
      p. ; cm.
   Includes bibliographical references and index.
   ISBN 978-1-59756-786-2 (alk. paper) — ISBN 1-59756-786-8 (alk. paper)
   I. Denti, Lou, author. II. Weber-Olsen, Marcia, author. III. Title.
   [DNLM: 1. Child Development Disorders, Pervasive—rehabilitation. 2. Child Development. 3. Education, Special—methods. WS 350.8.P4]
   RJ506.A9
   649'.154—dc23
                              2015034078

Contents

Introduction

Public schools have experienced a significant increase in the number of students qualifying for special education and related services under the disability category of Autism Spectrum Disorder (ASD). As a result, many states are developing additional certification or authorization in this area, which in turn is increasingly becoming a requirement for employment in teaching students with ASD in school districts. However, with or without additional certification, many educational professionals still lack sufficient training and/or experience in providing effective instruction and meaningful support to these students. Consequently, many educational professionals may feel overwhelmed when faced with the prospect of providing instruction to a population of students with unique challenges for whom they feel unprepared to teach. Fortunately, when considering this as a field, we have learned a number of things about how to provide educational supports to students with ASD within the context of real-world school and classroom settings. One of the things we have discovered is that simply delivering academic instruction is insufficient for this population. Rather, these students need to be provided with targeted and intentional interventions in the areas of interacting with others in the school's social context and in communicating effectively with others. Only when students with ASD are exposed to effective strategies supporting the development and active use of social-communicative skills with their peers and family members will we really begin to positively affect the overall quality of their lives.

Second, we have come to know through practical experience that supporting students with ASD in this way cannot be the responsibility of any single professional. These supports cannot be provided piecemeal by various disciplines working in isolation from one another. Instead, it truly takes a collaborative effort between those more experienced professionals willing to support and coach their fellow colleagues and those newer to this area, who must be willing to recruit input, ask for help, and tirelessly try out new ideas. Many school districts are currently providing beginning teachers with a more experienced colleague to serve as a coach by supporting the new teacher as he or she "learns the ropes." We feel that this type of a coaching arrangement can be a powerful opportunity for collaboration and skill building, ultimately benefitting students most of all.

The purpose of this book is to provide practitioners, including speech and language professionals, general and special education teachers, and other service providers with a resource to support their collaborative efforts to teach meaningful skills to students with ASD. The first section of the book presents a multitiered model for providing coaching at varying levels of support intensity, along with the numerous important considerations involved in implementing effective coaching supports. The second section of the book presents an outline of effective practices in utilizing coaching strategies to support teachers in planning for the instruction of meaningful skills to students with ASD utilizing a team-based, collaborative coaching model. The third section of the book provides numerous practical, evidence-based strategies to be used by coaches and teachers in teaching meaningful skills to students with ASD. We end the book with a chapter addressing critical issues involved in building the capacity of districts to evaluate, oversee, and support the effective coaching of teachers in providing evidence-based practices to students with ASD.

Acknowledgments

We wish to acknowledge all of the individuals with autism spectrum disorder (ASD), family members, educators, and related service providers with whom we have had the pleasure of working, teaching, and learning from. Without these meaningful relationships, and the willingness of these individuals to share their struggles, concerns, insights, and triumphs with us, this book would not exist.

We would also like to extend our gratitude to the editing team at Plural Publishing. We are especially grateful to Valerie Johns, Executive Editor, for her support and belief in this project. A special note of appreciation goes to Kalie Koscielak, Project Editor, for her extremely helpful guidance with regard to the many steps involved in taking a good idea all the way through to becoming a practical resource for educators. Last, we would like to thank Megan Carter, Production Manager, for her outstanding work with the final copyediting and designing the cover for this book.

SECTION I

High-Quality Coaching

Section I of this book provides the reader with a general background on educational coaching. We then provide information critical to educators in understanding the unique characteristics and needs of students with autism spectrum disorder (ASD). Next, coverage of useful models of coaching teachers in the development of best practices is provided. This is followed by a review of the essential roles and responsibilities coaches take on when supporting teachers to better serve students with ASD. The final chapter of this section introduces the High-Quality Coaching model of comprehensive coaching to support teachers of students with ASD, consisting of three specific coaching roles: peer-to-peer, consultative, and intensive coaching.

CHAPTER 1

Introduction to Educational Coaching

We must be the change we wish to see in the world.
—Gandhi

Chapter Objectives

- Describe trends related to educational coaching.

- Highlight the need for educational coaching in special education.

- Define coaching terms.

- Identify interpersonal and external variables that influence coaching.

- Identify the benefits of and obstacles to effective coaching.

- Set the terms for coaching engagement through high-quality coaching.

Trends in Educational Coaching

The Elementary and Secondary Education Act (ESEA, 2002) compelled changes to educational practices with the objective that student academic preparedness, achievement, and high school graduation rates in the United States increase going into the 21st century. As an outgrowth of this legislative mandate, educational consultation has been implemented in the public schools as a best practice for supporting teachers in the general education system (Kampwirth, 2006; Israel, Carnahan, Snyder, & Williamson, 2012). Educational consultation is designed to assist teachers and families in problem solving targeted academic interventions and positive behavior supports in the classroom before at-risk students fail academically and become disempowered. An exploration of the pedagogy of educational consultation suggests that although its research effectiveness is yet to be fully validated, the practice itself is here to stay and, in fact, has driven change in public schools for the better (Idol, 1990; Joyce & Showers, 2002). As in general education, the trend toward school-based consultation for students with special needs has been on the upswing (Cramer, 1998; Hanft, Rush, & Shelden, 2004; Israel et al., 2012). Consultation as a best practice in special education has been strongly influenced by mandates in the federal reauthorization of the Individuals with Disabilities Education Improvement Act (IDEIA, 2004) requiring public schools

to use scientifically based instructional practices to improve outcomes for children. A second component of IDEIA focused on facilitating training and use of personnel in the educational system to deliver instructional best practices in order to drive systemic change in the public schools. As a result, while not yet the norm, educational experts who support special education personnel are becoming more common in the public schools. The dramatic increase in the prevalence of autism spectrum disorder (ASD), a disabling handicapping condition affecting 1 in 68 in early childhood (U.S. Centers for Disease Control, 2010), and the demand for outcome-oriented interventions has driven the sea change in educational expectations for this disability. Autism spectrum disorder is a complex, neurodevelopmental condition that necessitates that personnel teaching students with this perplexing disability be well trained and prepared. Box 1–1 identifies the comprehensive knowledge and skills required by personnel who teach students with ASD based on the competency areas initially cited by Scheuermann, Webber, Boutot, and Goodwin (2003).

Special education teachers, now and in the future, need to implement evidence-based practices so that students make measurable academic and social progress. However, despite recognized national standards for educating children with ASD (National Research Council, 2001) as well as evidence-based practices disseminated by the National Autism Center (2009, 2015), educators have identified a "research to practice

Box 1–1. Knowledge and Skills
Required to Instruct Students With ASD

- Knowledge about the characteristics and core challenges of individuals with ASD

- Known and suspected etiologies of ASD

- Social communication and language characteristics of individuals with ASD

- Social communication teaching using evidence-based strategies

- Disparities in cognitive and adaptive abilities

- Socialization with peers

- Learning and motivation

- Behavior challenges and management

- Curriculum development in academic and functional skill acquisition

- Establishment of classroom structure and organization: routines, schedules, visual supports, and assistive technology

- Theoretical foundations of evidence-based intervention approaches

- Skill in delivering a range of evidence-based practices

- Assessment and data collection

- IEP writing

- Transition planning

- Working with parents

- Special issues: inclusion; teaming; managing related personnel, including instructional assistants (paraprofessionals); and in-home training

(Adapted from Scheuermann et al., 2003)

gap" in the delivery of scientifically validated interventions in classrooms for these students (McLeskey & Billingsley, 2008; Yell, Dragow, & Lowery, 2005). Other challenges include a shortage of a qualified and well-prepared teaching pool (Scheuermann et al., 2003); providing accommodations for Common Core standards; and ensuring that test-taking by students is not prioritized over meaningful instruction (Kretlow & Bartholomew, 2010). Resources are available for training educational personnel to effectively implement evidence-based approaches for students with ASD (see Section III); yet, multiple challenges persist in the preparation of personnel to instruct this population.

Definition of Terms

An *educational consultant* is someone responsible for guiding and supporting teachers to do more than implement teaching methods or accommodations appropriate to meet the needs of a particular student. A consultant enters into a relationship with one or more professionals who have recruited outside assistance and are willing to accept direction and support. Experts have described this process as collaborative, and it entails skill in nurturing "egalitarian" and "non-hierarchical" interpersonal relationships (Idol, Paoloucci-Whitcomb, & Nevin, 2000; Sheridan, Welch, & Orme, 1996). In this chapter, we further define the consultant as *mentor* and *coach*, and the *coachee* as the individual being coached. We envision a successful coach-coachee

experience as an ongoing, reciprocal relationship where problem solving and professional growth are the desired outcomes for teachers and educational staff in addition to improvement in student outcomes. Box 1–2 cites additional definitions of educational coaching from a cross section of publications on the topic.

As more educators and stakeholders, including parents and the court systems, take on the debate of what the federal law requires for the assurance of a "free and appropriate public education" (FAPE) for individuals with ASD, school agencies have utilized the expertise of consultants and coaches to ensure that FAPE occurs in the least restrictive educational setting. Even though instructional coaching can be conceptualized as best practice for serving this student population (Kucharczyk, Shaw, Smith Myles, Sullivan, Szidon, & Tuchman-Ginsberg, 2012), there are few resources to guide coaches and special educators on how to undertake this collaborative process successfully. Tables 1–1 and 1–2 identify some of the advantages as well as the realistic obstacles to the implementation of coaching. We return to a discussion of these obstacles later in this chapter as well as in the final chapter of this book.

Throughout the rest of this chapter, we address the need for educational coaching providing insight and case vignettes about students on the autism spectrum, teachers, and their classrooms experiences. This prompts further discussion of several key points about coaching. There are potential pitfalls or obstacles that teachers and special education teams can anticipate

Box 1–2. Definitions of Educational Coaching

- "A teacher receives initial preparation followed by ongoing individualized support from an expert mentor" (Kretlow & Bartholomew, 2010).

- Coaching is "concerned with drawing out solutions to problems by effective questioning and listening" (Allison & Harbour, 2009).

- "A coach provides ongoing embedded support and resources in a one-on-one relationship with a teacher" (Israel et al., 2012).

- "The goal of coaching teachers is to improve their use of a specific practice, such as the implementation of a program or general teaching skills" (Becker, Darney, Domitrovich, Keperling, & Ialongo, 2013).

when they engage with one another in the classroom. Communicative styles that resolve interpersonal conflict are one focus of this book in addition to a procedural framework for coaching teachers and all stakeholders in helping students succeed. This is not an intuitive process; coaching, like teaching, requires intentional planning and explicit practice for it to be worthwhile. However, the payoffs are potentially great when personnel are as taxed as

Table 1–1. Benefits of Coaching

Identified Benefit	Source
Improves teaching practices and professional satisfaction/self-efficacy over single workshop professional development	Israel, Carnahan, Snyder, & Williamson, 2012; Knight, 2007
Improves IEP outcomes	Ruble, Birdwhistell, Toland, & McGrew, 2011
Improves teacher retention; reduces professional burnout	Israel, Carnahan, Snyder & Williamson, 2012; Scheuermann, Webber, Boutot, & Goodwin, 2003
Improves fidelity of implementation of evidence-based practices by the teacher	Stahmer, Reed, Lee, Reisinger, Connell, & Mandell, 2015
Enhances collegiality among professionals	Eller & Eller, 2009

Table 1–2. Potential Obstacles to Coaching

Potential Obstacle	Source
Lack of enough expert personnel	Israel, Carnahan, Snyder, & Williamson, 2012
Time and financial resources to implement coaching suggestions in classrooms	Scheuermann, Webber, Boutot, & Goodwin, 2003
Strategies and resources to support coaching are lacking	McLeskey & Billingsley, 2008
Conflict with outside consultation agencies with differing ideologies	Scheuermann, Webber, Boutot, & Goodwin, 2003

they are in public education. The goal is not accomplishing more with less, but engaging in coaching with high quality. To do this well, district administrators will need to provide tangible resources and expert personnel where key stakeholders are actively involved. Critical district resources for supporting effective coaching practices are justified and discussed further in the last chapter of this book (see Chapter 13).

Working With Educators and Professionals Serving Students With Autism Spectrum Disorder

The coaching of general education teachers to support the special education student with ASD is a practice that is increasing with the rising prevalence of this disability in the general population, and as greater numbers of high-functioning students with ASD are included in general education settings. One rationale driving the emphasis on

coaching is the comprehensive manner in which support services for students with ASD need to be delivered in the public schools. Like the continuum of effective interventions required for serving students with ASD, school-based related services have evolved with best practices for this population. A majority of school speech-language pathologists (SLPs) surveyed have indicated that providing therapy outside of the general education classroom environment is the predominant manner in which they deliver direct therapeutic services to children with a variety of speech and communication disorders (Brandel & Frome Loeb, 2011); however, the unique needs of students with ASD have necessitated a change in this traditional model of service delivery. Therapeutic models in which the clinician/therapist provides push-in support within the general education classroom setting have become the standard for many students on the autism spectrum requiring explicit communication and social skills training (McGinty & Justice, 2007). Related support services may also be delivered through cotreatment by two or more therapists; for example, by the SLP and occupational therapist (OT) such that therapists' time is commonly spent in classroom settings where students spend the greatest part of their day. Depending on need, indirect support services may also be warranted where therapists consult with and support the educational team. National survey data collected by the American Speech-Language-Hearing Association (ASHA, 2012) show a majority (88%) of public school–based SLPs provide related services to students with an ASD diagnosis compared to a smaller percentage of those employed in public or private clinical settings. The average number of students with ASD on school SLP caseloads is 7.5 (ASHA, 2012).

Consultation and coaching are service options for teachers who can also benefit from the expertise of personnel from multiple disciplines skilled in working with students on the autism spectrum. Team-based support approaches are becoming common in public schools for serving students on Individualized Educational Programs (IEPs). Special and general education personnel along with related service providers and coaches may be involved in engineering learning and environmental supports as a student is integrated with typically developing peers in general education settings. Coaching requires an effective partnership with teachers and school personnel ensuring that IEP goals are implemented throughout the school day when the SLP or other personnel providing related servicers cannot be physically present with the student.

Finding Time and Resources for Coaching and Other Coaching Obstacles

Even though the concept of mentoring is generally regarded as a beneficial role relationship for both recipient and mentor, the coaching process in which an acknowledged expert provides oversight for someone in the role of novice can be a difficult undertaking. In educational settings, the novice learner—the beginning teacher or instructional assistant—is placed in an instructional role for which he or she is underprepared in some way. The coach is someone assumed to possess two essential skill sets: (a) the expertise and established knowledge about a subject area, and (b) the procedural and interpersonal skills needed to impart that knowledge effectively. Even though coaching would appear to be an ideal solution for teachers new to accommodating students with ASD, the implementation of it is often complicated by a number of issues within the typical educational setting, including teacher attitudes about inclusion, the status relationships of the coach and teacher, receptivity of the teacher to receiving performance feedback, not to mention prior years of teaching and coaching experience. Other challenges include ongoing professional development for teachers, coaches, and staff and the support systems that need to be in place for general education teachers to be successful with special education students included in their classrooms. Segall and Campbell (2012) have reviewed factors influencing teachers' and administrators' perceptions about inclusive education for students with ASD.

There is a need for collegial relationships in the coaching process to be established early on, although this component is often overlooked in busy school systems. Coaches who are assigned rather than recruited into a support role for a classroom teacher as done by Mr. Allison in the vignette (Box 1–3) can be extremely challenged in establishing effective working relationships with the teaching staff they consult with. The vignette in Box 1–4 depicts another realistic challenge.

Box 1–3. Vignette: "Just Do It" Coaching

Speech-Language Pathologist, Ms. Taylor, entered Brookings Elementary School excited about the upcoming year. Prior to her first day at school, she had met with the director of special education, learned about her caseload, and was relieved to know that she would not have to split her time between five schools. As she walked down the hallway, the principal, Mr. Townsend, told her in a rather abrupt manner that she would be coaching Mrs. LaGloria, the new third-grade teacher, on how to work with an autistic student she was getting in the next week from a school across town. As he hurried past, he said in a patronizing tone, "Ms. Taylor you're the expert in speech-language, and most students with autism have communication problems; you'll be a great help to Mrs. LaGloria." Just then a sixth grader bumped into Mr. Townsend, and he was off to other business. Ms. Taylor had zero knowledge and training in coaching other professionals and had minimal experience working side by side in a general education classroom. She had taken trainings offered by the district on strategies to work with students with ASD in the elementary grades. However, she felt like a neophyte in regard to working with this population and woefully unprepared to coach another teacher on how to best work with students with ASD in a general education classroom. Her excitement for the year had now turned to worrying about this new responsibility.

What is wrong with this picture? How should the principal have approached Ms. Taylor? Can we assume that because professionals are competent in their field of expertise that it automatically qualifies them to coach others?

Box 1–4. Vignette: "You Need It" Coaching

Mr. Allison, the principal at George Mason Middle School, has a reputation for going out of his way to interact positively with his staff. Sometimes, his upbeat style can be misinterpreted and teachers can take him the wrong way, as you will note in the following dialogue.

Mr. Allison: "Amy, we are finally getting you a coach after your experience with Rico last year. We know how hard it is to work with students with ASD, and we think that coaching will help you develop skills to work with Rico and your new student, Jordi. The coach is from the county office of education and is a friend of mine. She is busy, but she has a strong background in working with students with ASD. I know that Rico's parents can be a bit dominating from time to time, and your new coach will really help you understand how to deal with them. I have contacted her, and she is coming by my office next Tuesday. I will send her down to your class so she meets you, Rico, and Jordi. Make sure to introduce her to the IAs [instructional assistants] working with both kids. This is going to be great because these kids are not going away any time soon. Matter of fact, I read that autism is now an epidemic nationwide."

Amy: "Mr. Allison, I don't know if I am ready to have another person observing or helping me right now. I am swamped with other duties and feel that Rico and Jordi are doing just fine."

Mr. Allison: "Don't worry, Amy. It will be great and I think you will thank me in the long run."

What is wrong with this picture? Do you think Amy feels like she lacks the requisite skills to work with Rico and Jordi and needs corrective action? Mr. Allison's style of communication has left Amy feeling less than confident about an experience for which she has real trepidation.

Teachers must be willing to relinquish a portion of their classroom control to the coach, and the coach must be respectful of the teacher's flexibility in doing so. Experienced teachers in general education may be reluctant to implement accommodations that they perceive as violating uniform instructional standards for all students. In the same vein, teachers who feel imposed upon by school administrators anxious for the expertise of a specialist may harbor resentment about being coached. The unique needs of students with ASD further complicate the relationship between coach and coachee because of the wide variation in behavioral symptoms and individual learning strengths and weaknesses of students with this diagnosis.

Other demands for resources as well as planning time drive coaching outcomes. For example, visual learning supports for students with ASD, while readily available in self-contained settings, are resources that often must be reconstructed "on the fly" in inclusive settings. Time for follow-up consultation is rarely built into the school day, so that coaching often competes with other school activities and teacher obligations. Unique student needs and a multitude of personnel variables may combine to create the perfect storm in the general education classroom, where teachers and instructional assistants (paraprofessionals) may have little prior training knowing how to differentiate instruction for students. Additionally, coaches require ongoing training and resources to interact effectively with teachers and their staff and to be able to problem-solve the complex learning demands of students with ASD (McLeskey & Billingsley, 2008).

If we break down the coach-teacher relationship, it might be visualized as a dynamic process influenced by a number of factors illustrated in Figure 1–1.

Relationship building between coach and teacher evolves as a result of several interpersonal and extrapersonal variables. When these variables can be optimized, the impact on the student is positive and, in turn, results in favorable outcomes for teacher and coach. A successful coach is able to capitalize on those external factors that can be physically managed; for example, providing tangible supports in the classroom that enable student success. At the same time, the coach must accommodate the extrapersonal resources of the teacher, including his or her instructional skills and receptivity to coaching that influence the coach-teacher dynamic. This process is one of establishing rapport and trust, yet it also extends to role exchange for both teacher and coach. Effective coaching requires attuned skill at listening and deferring to the knowledge the teacher has to share about a student's preferences, strengths, habits, learning challenges, and uniqueness. Likewise, the teacher assumes a learner role with the coach who has expert knowledge about instructional strategies and ways of managing behavior. Once a teacher has demonstrated self-confidence in implementing effective strategies, a perceptive coach will step back from imparting ideas and consult from the sidelines, maintaining communication with the adult(s) now assuming a primary support role with the student. Chapter 4 elaborates on key attributes of effective coaching.

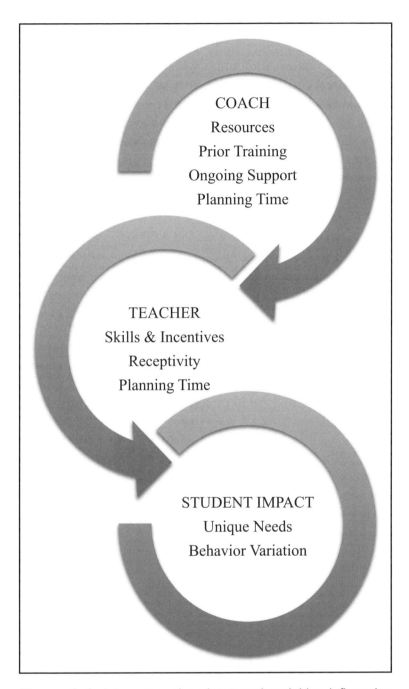

Figure 1–1. Interpersonal and external variables influencing coaching.

When students become successful, the impact of their learning increases the self-confidence of teaching staff as well as the likelihood that instructional success will be replicated with others who enter the classroom with similar challenges. A cycle of recursivity shown by the bidirectional arrows in Figure 1–1 occurs and increases the likelihood that teachers will develop autonomy and competence to serve future students. Early childhood intervention specialists have described similar consultative models for SLPs who coach parents in home settings to improve their young child's language development (Hanft et al., 2004; Woods, Wilcox, Friedman, & Murch, 2011).

There are essential features of the coaching process, including joint goal planning, self-reflection, systematic teaching with feedback, and problem solving that engender success (Woods et al., 2011). All of these interactive features are embedded in high-quality coaching. Another key component is ongoing professional development for educational staff, particularly new teachers. Educators have argued that one-time professional training consisting of lessons, demonstrations, and even practice and feedback is insufficient in impacting actual practice unless it is coupled with coaching with feedback in the classroom setting (Joyce & Showers, 2002). Data, in fact, indicate the ineffectiveness of single professional development inservice training in changing teaching practices for new teachers (Israel, Carnahan, Snyder, & Williamson, 2012).

High-Quality Coaching

Working with students on the autism spectrum can be, and often is, a joyful and rewarding experience. On the flipside, the challenges educators face teaching this population can be taxing and frustrating. The degree of difficulty for an educator working with students with this disability cannot be measured with a linear-type scale or assessment. The complexity of the assignment requires a great deal of pedagogical expertise. Providing expert coaching to help an educator learn about curricular and instructional best practices and then employ them with fidelity is paramount to career success. The right mentor or coach makes a major difference in how comfortable a teacher feels in fulfilling his or her role. Therefore, it is incumbent upon the coach to build relationships and to be fully aware of the educational context for a teacher or team in order to provide the most targeted support and guidance. Building a relationship takes time. The coach might find it difficult to establish meaningful contact as well as have occasion to discuss sensitive issues because of overriding factors such as classroom interruptions, IEP meetings, credentialing commitments, and mandatory trainings established by the central office or educational agency. It is imperative that the coach be patient, set up debriefing times to talk things over, listen closely to the teacher, and then establish an action plan that is manageable and doable.

Classes serving students with ASD usually incorporate a number of adults with different agendas. Some service delivery scenarios consist of as many students with ASD as adults in the room; for example, the teacher, two or more instructional assistants, an SLP and OT, two behavior technicians, and a behavior consultant hired from a private agency. In a case like this, the coach, who has the requisite expertise to work with the classroom teacher on curricular and instructional methods, finds him- or herself dealing with adult communication issues more often than not. The high number of adults in the classroom can make instruction difficult and awkward. Too many adults in a class can turn into exactly that: "too many." Coaches may find themselves in a mediation role when conflicts arise between adults. Conflict resolution in these instances turns out to be equally as important as coaching of skill building. It entails responsive and perceptive adult-to-adult communication so pivotal in managing a classroom of students with varying levels of need. The vignette in Box 1–5 illustrates the importance of responsible communication and how easily education for students with ASD can be jeopardized.

The vignette in Box 1–5 points out the unanticipated problems confronting educators working with students with ASD. Coaches in these types of situations need a full battery of interpersonal skills to deal with the communication dilemmas that arise in order to help teachers become and stay effective. Coaching teachers who work with challenging students requires that the coach have expert interpersonal skills. Establishing a strong and enduring collaborative relationship using key communication methods, and then imparting skills through actionable strategies is critical for success. In order that instruction is soundly implemented, data collected appropriately, and student progress monitored, skilled coaching of instruction cannot be underestimated. The following key points for high-quality coaching serve as a reminder of how to establish a meaningful coach-coachee relationship and emphasize important coaching attributes highlighted elsewhere in Chapter 4 and throughout this book.

Box 1–5. Vignette: Buyer's Remorse, the Case of "Too Many Is Too Many"

Susan, one of my university credential students, called me during the summer to tell me she was overjoyed because she had just landed the dream job of her life. Much to her surprise she was offered the job right on the spot. The administrator painted a rosy picture of the classroom with two great instructional assistants, two behavioral technicians, a school psychologist, outside consultants hired to provide additional training, and an SLP assigned three times a week for 2 hours. The administrator also said there would be additional support from adaptive physical education (APE) and occupational therapy (OT). As she hung up the phone giddy with joy, I truly hoped this would be Susan's dream job; however, a newly minted special education teacher managing so many adults in a classroom told me the opposite might be true.

One month into the school year I received another call from Susan. This time she was crying, telling me she was ready to quit because there are only six students in her class but sometimes as many as eight adults who do not listen to her and have their own agendas. She tearfully stated,

> The instructional assistants, who have been with the classroom for over six years disregard everything I say telling me that's not what they've done in the past, and that everything I suggest just won't work. At every turn they undermine my credibility and treat me with a kind of courteous restraint. Just because I am much younger than they are, it's no excuse to be treated in a rude, disrespectful manner. The behavior technicians just take data all day long looking for any miscue and then share the data with me in a very robotic fashion. The school psychologist, though funny, talks in front of the children, constantly telling me how busy he is and flits in and out of the classroom making minimal contact with me or the students. I love my SLP, who has now become a shoulder to lean on and a mentor, supporting me at my IEP meetings, teaching communication and social skills to students, and helping me with classroom management. The APE specialist and OT are very dedicated and upbeat and have been very supportive; however, when they take the kids out of the class, sometimes the students are more keyed up when they return. I am ready to quit and have told my principal who, in turn, told the special education director, who then assigned a program specialist to work with me. We have met twice, and she has some resources to offer, but once again seems too busy. I am desperate for assistance from someone who will help me with managing adults and assist me in building a repertoire of skills I need to be an effective teacher. I love my kids and would hate to leave them high and dry. Sorry to be so long-winded, monopolizing the conversation, but I needed to get this off my chest. When I interviewed I was so hopeful and, now, I am so discouraged.

High-Quality Coaching Key Points

- Establish trust with your coachee by listening closely to what is or might be a potential problem with students or other adults.

- Build your relationship over time and do not assume a "best buddy" interaction as it undermines your credibility as a coach and mentor.

- Be responsive with a clear idea in mind of how to support the teacher.

- Make the teacher part of the solution with you by establishing a nonhierarchical relationship.

- Establish a learning relationship style and be open to suggestions from the coachee.

- Set coaching objectives so that you and your coachee clearly understand in objective terms what needs to be accomplished.

- Establish a commitment to change.

In upcoming chapters in the book, the essential attributes of communication between a coach and teacher are covered, laying the foundation for a positive relationship to be established and sustained. In any collaborative enterprise, communication between parties takes center stage. One furtive glance communicated in the wrong way can often signal frustration or dismay. Estab-

lishing reciprocal communication so that both parties listen attentively and value one another's contributions alleviates misunderstanding and provides a context for problem solving. However, communication only goes so far; the coach and coachee must put a plan into action and strive for a degree of mastery to accomplish the plan. Accordingly, clear actionable steps to finding a solution must also be put into place. Too often, solving a problem is moored on the side of good intention with little implementation or closure. Instead, an action plan that operationalizes a real intention and a commitment to solve a problem, establish a routine, or learn a new strategy, elevates communication to solution finding and forward thinking.

End-of-Chapter Questions

1. Many people have never learned how to be effective mentors and coaches. Mentoring is not simply answering questions and giving advice, it requires a unique set of skills and practice. A coach/mentor needs to _____. Complete the sentence with several bullet points, and then share your response with a colleague.

2. Discuss an area drawn from personal experience or supposition that entails interpersonal or external variable(s) (see Figure 1–1) that could create potential obstacles between a coach and coachee.

3. Idol et al. (2000) described the coaching process as collaborative as it entails skill in nurturing "egalitarian" and "nonhierarchical" relationships. First, define *egalitarian* and *nonhierarchical*, and then in your own words describe a relationship you have developed with a coach who works with you. Is it egalitarian and nonhierarchical? If yes, explain in detail. If no, explain in detail. If you are not teaching in a classroom setting, then describe how you would establish an egalitarian and nonhierarchical relationship with a coach.

4. Speech-language pathologists and occupational therapists are often called upon to coach teachers working with students with ASD. Would you rather have them provide services in the classroom so you can learn from one another in real time? Or, conversely, do you prefer that they provide individual treatment at another room on campus and then consult and share instructional strategies? If you think providing services in the classroom trumps instruction in an alternate setting, then explain your reasoning. If you think instruction in an alternate setting is the best way to provide intensive services, explain your answer in detail. If you think both service delivery options are required, then provide a detailed rationale for your response.

5. Review the vignette in Box 1–5 "Buyer's Remorse: The Case of 'Too Many Is Too Many.'" Acting as coach in this scenario, use the High-Quality Coaching Key Points as a guide to communicate with the frustrated teacher in this vignette. Highlight the most important points from the High-Quality Coaching Key Points that you think are imperative in assisting this teacher, and then write a justification for your reasoning.

References

Allison, S., & Harbour, M. (2009). *The coaching toolkit: A practical guide for your school*. London, UK: Sage.

American Speech-Language-Hearing Association. (2012). *Schools Survey Report: SLP Caseload Characteristics Trends 1995–2012*. Retrieved from http://www.asha.org

Becker, K. D., Darney, D., Domitrovich, C., Keperling, J. P., & Ialongo, N. S. (2013). Supporting universal prevention programs: A two-phased coaching model. *Clinical Child and Family Psychology Review, 16*(2), 213–228.

Brandel, J., & Frome Loeb, D. (2011). Program intensity and service delivery models in the schools: SLP survey results. *Language, Speech, and Hearing Services in Schools, 42*, 461–490.

Cramer, S. F. (1998). *Collaboration: A success strategy for special educators*. Boston, MA: Allyn & Bacon.

Eller, J., & Eller, S. (2009). *Creative strategies to transform school cultures*. Thousand Oaks, CA: Corwin.

Fox, L., Hemmeter, M. L., Snyder, P., Perez Binder, D., & Clarke, S. (2011). Coaching early childhood special educators to implement a comprehensive model for promoting young children's social competence. *Topics in Early Childhood Special Educa*tion, *31*, 178–191.

Hanft, B. E., Rush, D. D., & Shelden, M. L. (2004). *Coaching families and colleagues in early childhood.* Baltimore, MD: Paul H. Brookes.

Idol, L. (1990). The scientific art of classroom consultation. *Journal of Educational and Psychological Consultation, 1*(1), 3–22.

Idol, L., Paoloucci-Whitcomb, P., & Nevin, A. (2000). *Collaborative consultation,* Austin, TX: Pro-Ed.

Israel, M., Carnahan, C. R., Snyder, K. K., & Williamson, P. (2012). Supporting new teachers of students with significant disabilities through virtual coaching: A proposed model. *Remedial and Special Education, 34*(4), 195–204.

Joyce, B., & Showers, B. (2002). *Student achievement through staff development.* Alexandria, VA: Association for Supervision and Curriculum Development.

Kampwirth, T. J. (2006) *Collaborative consultation in the schools: Effective practices for students with learning and behavior problems* (3rd ed.). Columbus, OH: Pearson Merrill Prentice-Hall.

Kretlow, A. G., & Bartholomew, C. C. (2010). Using coaching to improve the fidelity of evidence-based practices: A review of studies. *Teacher Education and Special Education, 33*(4), 279–299.

Kucharczyk, S., Shaw, E., Smith Myles, B., Sullivan, L., Szidon, K., & Tuchman-Ginsberg, L. (2012). *Guidance and coaching on evidence-based practices for learners with autism spectrum disorders.* Chapel Hill, NC: University of North Carolina, Frank Porter Graham Child Development Institute, National Professional Development Center on Autism Spectrum Disorders.

McGinty, A. S., & Justice, L. (2007). Classroom-based versus pull-out intervention: A review of the experimental evidence. *EBP Briefs, 1*, 1–14.

McLeskey, J., & Billingsley, B. S. (2008). How does the quality and stability of the teaching force influence the research-to-practice gap? *Remedial and Special Education, 29*, 293–305.

National Autism Center. (2009). *Evidence-based practice and autism in the schools: A guide to providing appropriate interventions to students with autism spectrum disorders.* Randolph, MA: Author.

National Autism Center. (2015). *Findings and conclusions: National standards project, phase 2.* Randolph, MA: Author.

National Professional Development Center on ASD. (2014). *Evidence-based practices for children, youth, and young adults with Autism Spectrum Disorder report.* Retrieved from http://autismpdc.fpg.unc.edu/node/19

National Research Council. (2001). *Educating children with autism.* Washington, DC: National Academy Press.

Ruble, L., Birdwhistell, J., Toland, M. D., & McGrew, J. H. (2011). Analysis of parent, teacher, and consultant speech exchanges and educational outcomes of students with autism during COMPASS consultation. *Journal of Educational and Psychological Consultation, 21*(4), 259–283.

Scheuermann, B., Webber, J., Boutot, E. A., & Goodwin, M. (2003). Problems with personnel preparation in autism spectrum disorders. *Focus on Autism and Other Developmental Disabilities, 18*, 197–206.

Segall, M. J., & Campbell, J. M. (2012). Factors relating to education professionals' classroom practices for the inclusion of students with autism spectrum disorders. *Research in Autism Spectrum Disorders, 6*, 1156–1167.

Sheridan, S. M., Welch, M., & Orme, S. F. (1996). Is consultation effective? A review of outcome research. *Remedial and Special Education, 17*(6), 341–354.

Stahmer, A. C., Reed, S., Lee, E., Reisinger, E. M., Connell, J. E., & Mandell, D. S. (2015). Training teachers to use evidence-based practices for autism: Examining procedural implementation fidelity. *Psychology in Schools, 52*(2), 181–195.

U.S. Centers for Disease Control and Prevention. (2010). *Identified prevalence of autism spectrum disorders.* ADDM Network 2000–2010. Retrieved from http://www.cdc.gov/ncbddd/autism/data.html

U.S. Centers for Disease Control and Prevention. (2014). Prevalence of autism spectrum disorder among children aged 8 years. Retrieved from http://www.cdc.gov/mmwr/preview/mmwrhtml/ss6302a1.htm?s_cid=ss6302a1_w

U.S. Department of Education. (2002). *A blueprint for reform: The reauthorization of the elementary and secondary education act.* Retrieved from http://www2.ed.gov/policy/elsec/leg/blueprint/publicationtoc.html

Woods, J. J., Wilcox, J. J., Friedman, M., & Murch, T. (2011). Collaborative consultation in natural environments: Strategies to enhance family-centered supports and services. *Language, Speech, and Hearing Services in Schools, 42*, 379–392.

Yell, M. L., Drasgow, E., & Lowery, K. A. (2005). No Child Left Behind and students with autism spectrum disorders. *Focus on Autism and Other Development Disabilities, 20*, 130–139.

CHAPTER 2

Autism Spectrum Disorder: What Effective Coaches and Teachers Need to Know

Autism is part of my child, it's not everything he is.
My child is so much more than a diagnosis.

—S. L. Coelho

Chapter Objectives

- Justify the importance of the coach as an expert resource for updating knowledge related to the neuroscience and complexity of autism spectrum disorder (ASD).

- Identify and explain the core deficits challenging children and individuals with ASD.

- Relate the core deficits to practical ways to support students in their school settings.

- Review best practices for educating children with ASD as they relate to the core deficits.

- Identify recent changes to the diagnosis and classification of ASD and related disorders.

- Discuss reasons for the research-to-practice gap challenging teachers' classroom implementation of best practices for students with ASD.

Introduction

In the vignette in Box 2–1, we get some perspective about the importance of shared understanding, and what needs to be communicated with teachers who instruct students with ASD. Even though many students with this diagnosis are successfully included in general education, there can be a lag in up-to-date knowledge that informs a teacher's understanding of this complex disorder. Consultants and professional trainers have the opportunity to convey insight about the challenges common to individuals with ASD as well as the variability and unique expressions of the

---

Box 2–1. Vignette: Up to Date

Jennifer, a teacher serving students with moderate to severe disabilities at Renown Central School, overhears a teacher complaining to other teachers in the faculty lounge about a student with ASD who is included in her class. The teacher does not mind the student coming to his class with a behavior support aide, but does not quite understand the behaviors the student displays, or what to do about them. The student always wants to sit in a particular seat and adjust his pencil, or anything movable on his desk in such a repetitive manner that it can be distracting. The teacher commented on the behavior: "Every day, he just keeps doing this thing of adjusting his pencil in the same spot on his desk, and I think it's bugging some of the other students. I don't want to say much because I know these kids do that sort of thing; you know you hear about it all the time: rocking, twirling, shouting out. I'm glad the behavior aide is there. But honestly, I'm not sure why the aide even allows that kind of behavior, and why he doesn't put a stop to it with this student."

Jennifer had just discussed some of the core deficits of ASD with a coach/consultant who had been providing additional support to her classroom. She was grateful to get current on the latest diagnostic definitions for the disorder and appreciated the coach/consultant explaining some of the new terminology to her, so she now had a better understanding of how to discuss some of these core deficits with her team. She felt comfortable approaching this teacher to share some of her current understanding of ASD.

disorder, but they can be challenged in communicating that information in practical ways to educational teams. Comprehensive training in the principles of treatment for ASD as well as ongoing supervised experiences, including coaching, are essential for teachers to acquire the practical skills needed for classroom mastery (Scheuermann, Webber, Boutot, & Goodwin, 2003). Having a high-quality coach to partner with educators to inform them about outcomes in research, including current diagnostic terminology and important changes to symptoms and diagnostic classification of ASD, is essential for building a team's competence in addition to applying state-of-the-art teaching practices.

The purpose of this chapter is to provide a framework of shared knowledge for both coaches and educators so that teams communicate effectively with one another and implement timely and effective educational interventions for their students. We start with a detailed review of the core deficits in ASD and how these, in turn, can interact to create a cascade of behavioral challenges. Several factors that contribute to the "research-to-practice" gap are examined as they apply to the rising prevalence of ASD as well as changes in diagnostic classification that differentiate ASD from other disorders. Review of best educational practices for serving children and older students with ASD is also undertaken as a means of establishing shared understanding and communication among coaches, educational teams, and families so that student success is achieved.

Core Deficits of Autism Spectrum Disorder

Autism spectrum disorder is characterized by "core" deficits, or common features shared by individuals with the diagnosis. Although ASD is a heterogeneous disorder, which means that behavioral symptoms will not be manifested identically in all individuals with the diagnosis, there are common challenges that they experience.

Social Communication

Social communication is a core deficit and a hallmark of the disorder (Dawson et al., 2004; Volkmar, Charawska, & Klin, 2005). Even though adaptive skills and intellectual competency may be assessed as average or above in those with higher-functioning ASD, social communication challenges persist in adulthood and challenge their peer relationships. Core deficits in this area may be evidenced by a significantly delayed onset of speech, or lack of speech in children with ASD. However, even for those with fluent expressive language skills and competence in vocabulary and syntax, many individuals with ASD may still have difficulty participating in conversational interactions that require topic shifting, taking listener perspective, and utilizing social conventions, such as nonverbal communicative gestures and body postures that support social interaction. In order to meet criteria for an ASD diagnosis in the area of social communication, the 5th edition of the *Diagnostic and Statistical Manual* of the American Psychiatric Association (APA, 2013) requires that persistent deficits be seen in social communication and social interaction across multiple settings in all three of the following areas: (1) deficits in social-emotional reciprocity such as abnormal social approach, failure of normal back-and-forth conversation, reduced sharing of interests, emotions, or affect, or failure to initiate or respond to social interactions; (2) deficits in nonverbal communicative behaviors used for social interaction, such as poorly integrated verbal and nonverbal communication, abnormalities in eye contact and body language or deficits in understanding and using gestures, or a lack of facial expressions and nonverbal communication; and (3) deficits in developing, maintaining, and understanding relationships, such as difficulties adjusting behavior to suit various social contexts, difficulties with imaginative play or making friends, or absence of interest in peers (APA, 2013, Autism Spectrum Disorder, 299.00; F84.0).

> *Whenever you speak to someone, you are presuming the two of you have a certain degree of familiarity which your words might alter. So every sentence has to do two things at once: convey a message and continue to negotiate that relationship.*
>
> —Steven Pinker

Sharing of affect and emotional states with partners may be impaired as part of a broader symptom of social communication deficit in ASD. As a result, the ability to socially "attune" to a conversational partner is compromised, and opportunities for continued practice of these related skills diminish as students enter middle and high school where their mastery is essential to fitting in socially. The American Speech-Language-Hearing Association breaks down difficulties with social communication, also referred to as *pragmatics* or the social use of language, into the following three areas (ASHA, 2015). First, difficulties may arise in using language for various purposes, such as in greeting others or making requests. Second, difficulties may occur when changes in language are expected due to changing situations, such as when speaking to peers versus adults or in providing context to a communicative partner unfamiliar with the conversation topic or details. Last, individuals with ASD may display challenges with the pragmatic use of language in the area of following the "unwritten" rules of conversation, such as turn taking, staying on topic versus shifting topics, proximity, use of facial expressions and eye contact, and so on.

Author John Elder Robison (2008), diagnosed with Asperger syndrome as an adult, recalled that after repeated failed interactions with peers in high school, he sought out adults as his primary conversational partners:

> My disjointed replies didn't bring the conversation to an abrupt halt. And grown ups explained things to me . . . Kids weren't so good at that. (p. 11)

Joint Attention

Social communication has been extensively studied in very young children with autism beginning with early interactions with their parents. Based on observational studies with infants and toddlers, researchers have argued that differences in *social orienting* and *joint attention* underlie the core deficit in social communication (Dawson et al., 2004; Wetherby, Watt, Morgan, & Shumway, 2007). Joint attention occurs within a social context and entails the ability to coordinate attention between objects or events in interaction with a partner (Dawson et al., 2004). By definition, joint attention is *reciprocal* as it involves initiating and responding through a variety of social communicative means: alternating of eye gaze and turning the head in the same direction of a partner; following a gestural point of a partner; and/or directing the partner's attention through vocalization, gesture, and/or sharing of emotional state. The developmental trajectory of joint attention in toddlers with autism looks different from the typically developing child as well as from children with other developmental disabilities. Studies examining joint attention in infants and toddlers point to the importance of this capacity as a strong predictor of language development. Adamson and colleagues (Adamson, Bakeman, Deckner, & Romski, 2009) coded the onset of joint interaction in three toddler groups, including children with autism and Down syndrome, and found that even though toddlers in the ASD group surpassed the expressive and receptive language skills of those with Down syndrome, they had persistent deficits in the manner in which they coordinated joint attention in play with their mothers. In this study, children in the autism spectrum group were able to focus on a shared object (such as a wind-up toy) and were able to respond to language support from their mothers, yet had significantly more difficulty than did the toddlers with Down syndrome managing shared attention, using gaze shifts, securing the attentional focus of their mothers by looking at their line of regard, and initiating and responding in back-and-forth exchanges.

Research has pointed to impaired imitation skills as the root cause of deficits in joint attention, affect, and emotional sharing in autism. Imitation is the primary means by which the social culture is transmitted (Rogers, Bennetto, McEvoy, & Pennington, 1996). Rogers and colleagues found that in autism, the mimicking of facial and gestural movement patterns is evident but "muted in volume." This study found that imitation deficits continue into adolescence for individuals with high-functioning autism and are disparate from their stronger symbolic capacities for language. Fortunately, children with ASD do show significant improvement in joint attention, imitation, and social engagement when interventions systematically target these core deficits in early childhood (Kasari & Patterson, 2012; Wetherby et al., 2007). Patten and Watson (2011) identified 12 therapeutic intervention strategies focused on improving joint attention in children with autism, entailing child-directed play, reinforcement, adult imitation of the child's facial expressions, actions and/or gestural behavior, and cuing strategies. Their study found that targeting social imitation, joint attention, and sharing of emotions in a synchronous fashion over a 6-month duration with toddlers as young as 21 months of age had a significant improvement on their social communication and language skills, and their ability to generalize these skills to new people and settings.

Symbol Use

Social communication also entails the emergence of *symbols,* a milestone that manifests developmentally in a child's use of communicative gestures, symbolic play, and expressive-receptive language. Children with ASD may go on to establish a fascination with certain symbol forms, for example, letters, numbers, and words, yet they demonstrate qualitative differences in their acquisition and understanding of conventional social gestures and utilization of conventional meanings for words that map to language (Woods & Wetherby, 2003). Many who eventually acquire speech go through a stage of using echoic scripts to communicate long before they are able to use language in some spontaneous, rule-based fashion.

One landmark of symbol use is the developmental emergence of *symbolic* (pretend) *play.* Symbolic play in children with autism has been documented as qualitatively different from typically developing children (Rogers, 2000). Children with ASD are more likely to have fixated interests; consequently, their spontaneous play can be repetitive and limited to a preferred set of toys and a small set of repetitive actions on those items (e.g., banging, lining up). When a repetitive action scheme is employed again and again, it can restrict the child's problem solving and the emergence and progression of higher forms of symbolic play. Likewise, among higher-functioning older children with conversational skill, there may be a narrow set of intense interests that drive their topics in conversation; this is likely to restrict their social acceptance by peers who may become intolerant of this pattern.

Early joint attention is critical for the acquisition of symbol use as the child matures, because this skill is embedded in the social context of conversation. Shared attention is important for comprehending the communicative intentions of others and for modifying what is said based on the perspectives of one's social partners. Rubin and Lennon (2004) have detailed the vulnerabilities of older students with higher-functioning autism in joint attention and symbol use. As these authors point out, without the ability to secure the attentional focus of a partner and to accurately "perceive other's intentions and emotional states," students with ASD are at risk of social isolation. In contrast, typically developing children develop and employ joint attention and symbol use in sophisticated ways; this includes the ability to use social conventions when initiating and ending conversations as well as repairing communicative breakdowns by considering "plausible causal factors" for the emotional reactions of their conversational partners (Rubin & Lennon,

2004). Often referred to as perspective taking, this latter capacity to understand and be sensitive to a conversational partner's reactions to what is said is dependent on an ability to infer attributes of a partner's mental state and his or her feelings, beliefs, and intentions (Baron-Cohen, 1995). Perspective taking is an exceptionally challenging skill for individuals with higher-functioning ASD given their inherent difficulty with other aspects of social monitoring in dynamic interactions.

Repetitive and Restrictive Patterns of Behavior, Interests, and Activities

Core deficits in repetitive and restricted patterns of behavior, interests, and activities are also apparent in individuals diagnosed with ASD. Deficits related to repetitive and restricted patterns of behavior, interests, and activities manifest in a number of different ways, varying greatly from one individual to another. However, the *DSM-5* includes four distinct ways in which these restricted, repetitive patterns may be displayed (Note: According to the *DSM-5*, in order to meet diagnostic criteria for ASD in this area, impairments in at least two of the four areas would need to be apparent.) The first symptom area involves stereotyped, repetitive motor movements, use of objects, or speech. These may consist of motor stereotypy (e.g., repetitive hand movements), lining up objects, echolalia (e.g., repeatedly using the same words or phrases, or repeating the last word or phrase spoken by oth-

ers), and so on. The second symptom area is an insistence on sameness, inflexible adherence to routines, or ritualized patterns of verbal/nonverbal behavior. Examples in this area include extreme distress at small changes, difficulties with transitions, rigid thinking patterns, greeting rituals, needing to take the same route, or eating the same food every day. The third area entails highly restricted, fixated interests that are abnormal in intensity or focus. These include a strong attachment to, or preoccupation with unusual objects and obsessive interests. The last symptom area consists of hyper- or hyporeactivity to sensory input or unusual interests in sensory aspects of the environment. These can manifest as a seemingly indifferent response to pain or temperature, adverse responses to specific sounds or textures, excessive smelling or touching of objects, or a visual fascination with lights or movement (American Psychiatric Association, 2013).

Understandably, the core deficits in ASD interact with and complicate the interrelationship of one skill modality with another. For example, communicative frustration can result in a cascade of severe behavioral challenges. Students with ASD who are limited in their ability to use language may adopt idiosyncratic behavioral means of communicating via tantrums, physical aggression, and/or self-injurious behavior. Teachers and coaches play a crucial role in accurately interpreting and responding to those behaviors in the student. Adult partners can engage in functional behavioral assessment practices to determine the reason for, or function of, the behavior and respond with multicomponent behavior supports. (This approach is detailed in Chapter 11.) Teachers and coaches can also "engineer" environmental supports for those whose verbal language capacities are limited; for example, providing social narratives (written scripts) to recall the steps to calm down, or a location in the classroom that the student can access in order to relax and regroup. It is equally important for educators and coaches to be aware of particular environmental triggers that predict disruptive patterns of behavior in a student (e.g., transitioning to new activities, or encountering events and settings at school that typically overwhelm the student, such as the cafeteria or a fire drill). Teachers with support from their coaches can anticipate situations of anxiety and frustration in order to preempt environmental triggers and provide successful supports for the student. We see in the scenario presented in Box 2–2 how a student is unable to manage frustration, and a teacher's attempts to understand the source of the student's challenging behavior.

The vignette, "When Communication Fails," highlights a teacher's awareness regarding repetitive and restricted behaviors associated with students with ASD, a good first step. She also senses when Monique is ready to bolt. Her openness to coaching and support shows that she really wants to tackle this issue. This scenario may be an opportunity for consultative coaching. The coach would first want to make sure that the teacher does not feel like she is doing something wrong or causing the problem. The coach would want to spend time observing Monique's behavior in the classroom and engage the teacher and staff in a functional assessment process to determine the variables involved in Monique's bolting behavior. In this collaborative approach, the coach can put the teacher at ease listening closely for clues about the influences of the environment on Monique's behavior. Once the coach and teacher develop an initial rapport, they can begin to search for solutions. The coach may want to ask the teacher if she thinks addressing some classroom factors would give insight to Monique's bolting behavior. Teacher and coach would then review daily activity routines, schedules, and social interactions that may trigger or maintain Monique's behavior. They also may want to explore ways to support Monique's means of functional communication, and create opportunities for her to make choices so that academic tasks do not frustrate her. Rather than only trying to figure out when Monique is going to take off and what to do when this happens, a support plan can be developed with prevention also in mind. The support plan would need to involve all stakeholders, including staff, related service providers, parents, and others who work with Monique. One strategy could involve developing a simple weekly grid that divides the day up into half-hour blocks with choice-making opportunities offered every 30 minutes so that Monique learns the "power" of initiating communication with adults (e.g., by being offered regular intervals of time at a preferred activity). The school speech-language pathologist (SLP) should also be consulted about an augmentative-

Box 2–2. Vignette: When Communication Fails

Eleven-year old Monique is an enigma in my class. Her verbal skills are limited to two- or three-word phrases, pointing at symbols, understanding functional words like "stop," "no," "more," and "go," and using facial expressions that let us know if she is happy or displeased. She can be the most endearing person in the world and the most troublesome, because she suddenly bolts out of the class faster than the comic hero, Flash. The class then moves into lockdown mode with the instructional assistants mobilized to try and find her, the principal and all custodial and playground staff alerted, and the police contacted when she has eloped from campus. When Monique bolts it is serious business and, as you can imagine, nerve racking. When she is located and brought back to school, the staff, though relieved, are emotionally spent, and the rest of the day is a wash out. Monique runs off about twice a month.

I am keenly aware that this behavior may have a purpose to it, but I am flummoxed by the behavior and in dire need of support and guidance. The district keeps sending professionals to my classroom just after an incident happens to help me offset Monique's bolting behavior. These brief visits do little to assuage my fears; the plans are of little value, although they seem to assure the district office that something is being done. I know part of the reason Monique bolts is because she is unable to communicate her needs. I can sense when she is ready to make a dash for it, but I have yet to figure out how to stop it. I would like a mentor or coach to help me with this situation, develop an action plan, and then, at the very least, follow up with me throughout one semester so whatever is worked out is sustained not only for me, but also for the substitute teacher if I happen to be gone on a particular day.

alternative communication (AAC) evaluation to determine appropriate AAC communication supports for Monique that may affect a change in her behavior. This might entail use of an appropriate speech-generating device that would augment Monique's limited expressive output so that the rate of her communicative requests is increased during these shorter instructional blocks. Eventually, it would be essential to embed use of the AAC strategies in activities throughout Monique's school day.

Addressing Core Deficits in School Settings

How are interventions for social communication deficits best implemented in public school settings? Among several intervention guidelines recommended by the National Research Council (NRC, 2001), a focus on spontaneous functional communication was found to strongly predict best outcomes for children with ASD in several model intervention programs across the United States. Table 2–1 lists additional conditions satisfying best practice for instructing students with ASD.

Summative findings from the National Standards Project (National Autism Center, 2015) and the National Profes-

Table 2–1. Components of Instructional Best Practice for Students with ASD

1. Individualized interventions to adjust for the wide range of a given child's strengths and weaknesses
✓ Treatment must be highly individualized to child's unique needs
2. Focus on *spontaneous, functional communication* for all children with ASD and at all levels of disability
3. Child engaged in meaningful, functional learning activities that are motivating and developmentally appropriate
4. Naturalistic teaching approaches that begin with child choice and use functional and direct reinforcers to foster motivation and generalization
5. Well-defined set of teaching plans for developing functional skills, delivered at a high frequency throughout the day
6. Ongoing monitoring of progress and adjustment of teaching practices and content to maximize progress
7. Focus on the ecological validity of skills being taught and their maintenance and generalization in *functional daily routines* in natural settings and with multiple partners
8. Planned interactions with typically developing peers—crucial for social growth
9. Families actively involved in their children's treatment program
✓ Setting goals and priorities for their child's treatment
✓ Locating supports for themselves
✓ Supporting their child's new skills in home and community activities
✓ Receiving training in effective ways of teaching their children to function in family and community routines
10. Well-trained and prepared educational staff

Source: National Research Council: *Educating Children with Autism*, 2001.

sional Development Center for Autism Spectrum Disorder (Wong et al., 2014) also point to the importance of utilizing evidence-based practices to address social communication and repetitive and restricted patterns of behavior, interests, and activities in meaningful activities and routines within the school day. Teachers and school-based SLPs can collaborate on social communication goals to be targeted for improvement with intervention provided in typically occurring play routines with the child's preferred interests and toys, utilizing sensory materials and routines that increase joint engagement, and in simple back-and-forth exchanges that encourage shared interest, mutual gaze, and turn-taking. For older students, core deficits in social communication should be addressed through treatment strategies that facilitate social interaction, including practice in conversational exchanges with peers and other social partners. Similarly, teachers can collaborate with related service providers to provide behavior supports in typical school activities and routines to address core deficits in the areas of restrictive and repetitive patterns of behavior, interests, and activities. These topics will be a focus in Section III when we return to a discussion of evidence-based interventions.

Learning about and fully understanding the core deficits of ASD can be a daunting task for teachers stretched for time and resources. Those challenged by students exhibiting ongoing and intense difficulties at school certainly benefit from the expertise of someone with coaching experience. Nevertheless, sometimes coaches miss the mark, even when they are exceptionally well informed about educational best practices, as seen in Box 2–3.

Box 2–3. Vignette: Alphabet Soup

"Hello, I am Mrs. Smith, your coach hired by the school district. I don't think we've met, but I am here to help you with your students. My focus is in DTT and PRT, two evidence-based approaches to support students with ASD. So, I will do an observation today, take notes, and discuss how to implement these wonderful approaches. I am sure you've heard about DTT and PRT in your credential program, or from in-service training through your school district. I see you are keeping data on your students' behaviors and have recently been implementing DRO and DRA—or was it DRI?—with a few of your students, and that's a good thing. However, I will give you some new ways to provide instruction and address student behavior. Let me get started observing because my time is limited today. Just go about your day as usual."

As we see in this vignette, it is important that coaches do not assume prior knowledge of their consultees by using jargon that fails to effectively communicate. Although coaches ultimately must be willing to challenge beliefs and, if necessary, have difficult conversations with their consultees (Allison & Harbour, 2009), a solutions-focused approach will go further in ensuring that information is shared meaningfully. Interpersonal and communication characteristics are essential for successful coaching. Chapter 4 undertakes discussion of those attributes considered critical to optimal coaching outcomes with teachers and other stakeholders.

Diagnostic Updates and Current Issues: The Research-to-Practice Gap

The scenario in Box 2–3 illustrates a critical issue that teachers and ASD educational teams have experienced, or may eventually encounter, with regard to the terminology or professional jargon that is taken for granted as shared knowledge by experts who consult in their classrooms. Consulting agencies and coaches can make wrong assumptions about the background knowledge of teachers with limited resources for updating their skills about evidence-based instructional methodologies. Even among veterans in special education, the gap may be vast between a teachers' knowledge of theory and pedagogy about ASD and implementation of cur-

rent classroom practices. We previously emphasized this research-to-practice gap in Chapter 1 as a primary challenge for educators and administrators focused on quality programming for their students. Several factors contribute to this disparity between leading educational research and instructional delivery to the ASD population. Among the primary reasons is the rising prevalence of students with ASD and the capacity, or lack thereof, of school districts to accommodate the number of students with this disability. Agency and government statistics indicate that ASD in the United States increased 119.4 percent from the year 2000 when the incidence was reported at 1:150 (Centers for Disease Control and Prevention [CDC], 2015). Recent data show that 1 in every 68 children up to the age of 8 years will have a diagnosis of ASD in the United States, and among males the incidence is higher: 1 in 42 (CDC, 2015). Although ASD does not occur at lower rates among minority children, Travers, Krezmien, Mulcahy, and Tincani (2014) found that the prevalence of ASD diagnosis and Individualized Education Program (IEP) service provisions in public schools varied sharply among ethnic/racial groups. Latino and black students were far less likely to be identified and receive services than white children over a span of two reporting periods between 2000 and 2007. Clearly, challenges persist in school systems as a result of the sharp increase in the number of students qualifying under the federal disability category for autism. Local education agencies are taxed with keeping up with latest advances as well as finding qualified personnel and providing resources for more students who require a continuum of comprehensive treatment.

A second reason for the research-to-practice gap is the breadth and depth of knowledge needed to keep up with the increasing amount of research being conducted related to ASD and effective practices to support individuals with this disability. There has been an explosion of terminology commensurate with the upsurge of scientific findings and diagnostic changes related to this complex disorder. In 2013, the American Psychiatric Association updated its diagnostic classification of autism and related disorders in the *Diagnostic and Statistical Manual of Mental Disorders*, fifth edition (*DSM-5*), clarifying the diagnosis and providing description of core behavioral symptoms utilizing a set of broad principles to account for the heterogeneity of symptoms across the life span, cultural-social contexts, and functioning of individuals affected by ASD. Changes to the *DSM-5* clarified ambiguous and overlapping symptoms for Pervasive Developmental Disorders (PDD), which included autism, that appeared in the 1994 text revision (*DSM-IV TR*); PDD subgroups have been reconceptualized along a single continuum now called Autism Spectrum Disorder (ASD). What was once three domains of symptom involvement (language and communication, social relatedness, and restricted repetitive and stereotyped behavior) has now been simplified to two core domains in the *DSM-5*: social communication and restricted, repetitive patterns of behavior or interests. Delayed language acquisition and a failure to use verbal language are also no longer part of ASD criteria, as these symptoms are not exclusive to ASD. Rather, social communication symptoms for a diagnosis of ASD now include (a) social-emotional reciprocity, (b) nonverbal communicative behaviors used for social interaction, and (c) development, maintenance, and understanding of social relationships and adjustment of communication and behavior to suit various social contexts (Lord & Bishop, 2015).

A severity metric is included based on the intensity of supports required by individuals who receive the ASD diagnosis in the *DSM-5*. For example, a student who displays marked deficits even with substantial supports in place is categorized at a moderate level of severity (Level 2), while those with more severe symptom involvement are categorized at a Level 3 (Figure 2–1). It is important to note that severity ratings are used for descriptive purposes and not to diagnose or determine eligibility for services (American Psychiatric Association, 2013).

Although the diagnostic category for Asperger syndrome is now eliminated from the autism spectrum, the *DSM-5* differentiates a new diagnostic category for a "social communication (pragmatic) disorder" in which the scope of symptoms differs from ASD (Figure 2–2). Restricted, repetitive behaviors are not witnessed in SCD, and symptoms are not otherwise accounted for by intellectual disability or general language delay (Lord & Bishop, 2015). Thus, an ASD

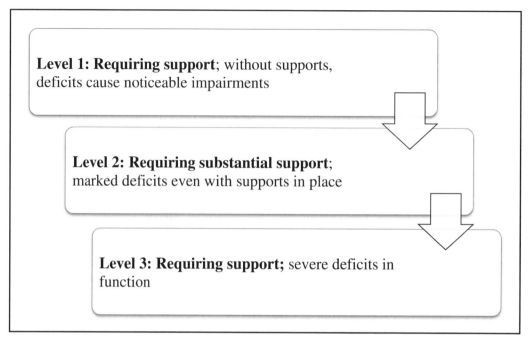

Figure 2–1. Severity and levels of support related to ASD (American Psychiatric Association, 2013).

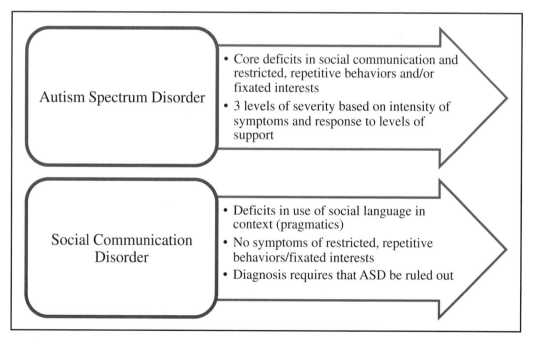

Figure 2–2. Diagnostic distinctions between ASD and social communication disorder (American Psychiatric Association, 2013).

diagnosis must first be ruled out before SCD is confirmed. A discussion of social communication disorder as it relates to assessment issues appears in Section II of this book (see Chapter 7).

Consequences of the research-to-practice gap can be painfully evident when there is disagreement among parents and other members on the IEP team. This is particularly true when methodologies used in a preschool or school program are not consistent with treatment and service plans for children transitioning to an IEP in schools, or for those students transferring from elsewhere in the country with IEPs in hand. Educational agencies must be prepared to deliver defensible IEPs, which necessitates a program of instruction that follows the free and appropriate public education (FAPE) standard and aligns with best practice guidelines for instructing children with ASD. Yell and Drasgow (2000) have emphasized that a majority of legal challenges by parents contesting implementation of IEPs was largely due to a lack of comprehensive programming and training of school personnel. Although some progress has been made to this end, teachers are still faced with the dilemma of responding to parents insisting on a specific intervention program to the exclusion of broader instructional approaches that address a child's primary challenges. As previously discussed, core deficits in spontaneous communication and social interaction can be especially resistant to change in ASD and will require interventions that may require significant training and professional development in order to be implemented with fidel-

ity (i.e., correctly). Having a comprehensive foundation of knowledge and practical skills ensures that teachers will be able to educate parents who embrace a single ideology, or intervention methodology, and those who may be too eager to adopt an untested "bandwagon" approach to treatment. Having a breadth of teaching methods based on scientifically validated practices can effectively address the core deficits seen among students with ASD and additionally, avoids the misconception that "one-size-fits-all" in which rigid adherence to a single methodology can prevail in classrooms. Guidelines specified by the NRC (2001) for educating children with ASD argue strongly against exclusive reliance on only a single evidence-based practice. In Section III we return to a discussion of evidence-based interventions for ASD that satisfy the standard for varied instructional approaches and focused interventions appropriate for addressing the unique needs of students with ASD.

Summary

In this chapter an overview of ASD and its common, or core, deficits were provided. Social communication and its related components of joint attention, symbol use, and pragmatics are primary challenges in the disorder, beginning in early development and persisting well into adolescence and adulthood. Even though verbal language skills emerge and become sophisticated among many with higher-functioning abilities, social communication deficits have a cascading effect on the social competence of individuals affected with ASD. Restricted and repetitive behavior, interests, and activities are also persistent core deficits, although symptom presentation varies widely both across individuals and across the life span of individuals with ASD.

Recent changes to the diagnostic classification system have clarified important distinctions between an ASD diagnosis and related language disorders as they appear in the updated *DSM-5*. Understanding the current characteristics associated with ASD is important for effectively addressing many of the unique behavioral symptoms that individuals with ASD demonstrate, and coaches play a critical role in imparting this information to educational teams. Parents need up-to-date information about the breadth of evidence-based supports available for their child with ASD so that unhelpful, or even dangerous, ideologies and methodologies do not prevail. Having a teacher who is well coached in current practices and in the characteristics of ASD ensures the best educational outcomes.

End-of-Chapter Questions

1. List and explain the core deficits that characterize autism spectrum disorder.

2. As a teacher of a special education program that services students with ASD, how would you explain the core deficit of restricted and repetitive patterns of behavior, interests, and activities to a parent of a child with this challenge?

3. How do the core deficits interact with each other in ASD? Give an example from a student with whom you are familiar, or identify a case example in this textbook.

4. Explain the research-to-practice gap as it applies to classrooms that serve students with ASD.

5. As a future expert coach, what information do you regard as essential for educational staff and teachers to know and understand about helping students with ASD?

6. What is the difference diagnostically between ASD and social communication disorder? What service providers will be important to assist with this diagnosis?

7. Assume you are a teacher in a classroom for elementary students with ASD. What educational guidelines will you want to focus on to ensure that you are implementing standards of best practice for your students?

8. Respond to question #7 above, assuming your students are in middle or high school.

References

Adamson, L. B., Bakeman, R., Deckner, D. F., & Romski, M. (2009). Joint engagement and the emergence of language in children with autism and Down syndrome. *Journal of Autism and Other Developmental Disorde*rs, *39*(1), 84–96.

Allison, S., & Harbour, M. (2009). *The coaching toolkit: A practical guide for your school.* London, UK: Sage.

American Psychiatric Association. (2013). *Diagnostic and statistical manual of mental disorders* (5th ed.). Washington, DC: Author.

American Speech-Language-Hearing Association. (2015). *Social language use (pragmatics).* Retrieved July 16, 2015, from http://www.asha.org/public/speech/development/Pragmatics.htm

Autism Society of America. (2015). *Facts and statistics.* Retrieved July 16, 2015, from http://www.autism-society.org/what-is/facts-and-statistics/

Baron-Cohen, S. (1995). *Mind blindness: An essay on autism and theory of mind.* Boston, MA: MIT Press.

Centers for Disease Control and Prevention. (2015). *Autism Spectrum Disorder: Data and statistics.* Retrieved July 16, 2015, from http://www.cdc.gov/ncbddd/autism/data.html

Dawson, G., Toth, K., Abbott, R., Osterling, J., Munson, J., Estes, A., & Liaw, J. (2004). Early social attention impairments in autism: Social orienting, joint attention, and attention to distress. *Developmental Psychology, 40*(2), 271–283.

Kasari, C., & Patterson, S. (2012). Interventions addressing social impairments in autism. *Current Psychiatry Reports, 14*(6), 713–725.

Lord, C., & Bishop, S. L. (2015). Recent advances in autism research as reflected in DSM-5 criteria for autism spectrum disorder. *Annual Review of Clinical Psychology, 11*, 53–70.

National Autism Center. (2015). *Findings and conclusions: National standards project, phase 2.* Randolph, MA: Author.

National Research Council. (2001). *Educating children with autism.* Washington, DC: National Academy Press.

Patten, E., & Watson, L. R. (2011). Interventions targeting attention in young children with autism. *American Journal of Speech-Language Pathology, 20*, 60–69.

Robison, J. E. (2008). *Look me in the eye! My life with Asperger's.* New York, NY: Crown.

Rogers, S. J. (2000). Interventions that facilitate socialization in children with autism. *Journal of Autism & Other Developmental Disorde*rs, *30*(5), 399–409.

Rogers, S. J., Bennetto, L., McEvoy, R., & Pennington, B. F. (1996). Imitation and pantomime in high-functioning adolescents with autism spectrum disorders. *Child Development, 67*(5), 2060–2073.

Rubin, E., & Lennon, L. (2004). Challenges in social communication in Asperger syndrome and high-functioning autism. *Topics in Language Disorders, 24*(4), 271–285.

Scheuermann, B., Webber, J., Boutot, E. A., & Goodwin, M. (2003). Problems with personnel preparation in autism spectrum disorders. *Focus Autism and Other Developmental Disorders, 18*, 197–206.

Travers, J. C., Krezmien, Mulcahy, C., & Tincani, M. (2014). Racial disparity in administrative autism identification across the United States during 2000 and 2007. *Journal of Special Education, 48*, 155–166.

Volkmar, F., Charawska, K., & Klin, A. (2005). Autism in infancy and early childhood. *Annual Review of Psychology, 56*, 315–336.

Wetherby, A. M., Watt, N., Morgan, L., & Shumway, S. (2007). Social communication profiles of children with autism spectrum disorders late in the second year of life. *Journal Autism and Other Developmental Disorders, 37*, 960–975.

Woods, J., & Wetherby, A. (2003). Early identification of and intervention for infants and toddlers who are at risk for autism spectrum disorder. *Language, Speech, and Hearing Services in Schools, 34*, 180–193.

Wong, C., Odom, S. L., Hume, K. Cox, A. W., Fettig, A., Kucharczyk, S., & Schultz, T. R. (2014). *Evidence-based practices for children, youth, and young adults with Autism Spectrum Disorder.* Chapel Hill, NC: University of North Carolina, Frank Porter Graham Child Development Institute, Autism Evidence-Based Practice Review Group.

Yell, M. L., & Drasgow, E. (2000). Litigating a free appropriate public education: The Lovaas hearings and cases. *Journal of Special Education, 33*, 205–214.

CHAPTER 3

Educational Coaching:
A Review of Models
and Methods

*I think a role model is a mentor—someone you see
on a daily basis, and you learn from them.*

—Denzel Washington

Chapter Objectives

■ Provide an overview of peer-based and expert coaching
models in the educational literature.

■ Describe coaching models and activities utilized with
teachers who instruct students with autism spectrum
disorder (ASD).

■ Evaluate the benefits of coaching relative to student,
teacher, and family outcomes.

■ Introduce information on alternative methods of
coaching delivery utilizing technology.

Introduction

When it comes to training teachers to implement effective instruction and behavior support, coaching is essential. Joyce and Showers (2002) provide a breakdown of the extent to which knowledge of content, skill demonstration, and classroom application by teachers occurs in response to various training components. The training components evaluated include presentation/lecture, demonstration, practice, and coaching with feedback (with administrative support for this activity). As seen in Table 3–1, only when the coaching component is provided, in addition to the other training components, do teachers reach a level of competency in all three training outcomes (Joyce & Showers, 2002).

For decades educators and researchers have attempted to identify the essential elements of effective educational coaching (Joyce & Showers, 1982; Koegel, Russo, & Rincover, 1977). Various authors have examined models of coaching and how they can be successfully implemented (for a review see Denton & Hasbrouck, 2009). This chapter begins with an overview of coaching models, including peer-based models, in which teachers take turns demonstrating and observing an instructional method, and expert models, in which someone with substantial knowledge of a pedagogical approach imparts that information to someone less experienced in it. We review coaching models developed for the general education setting and proceed to those studies examining coaching in special education and, in particular, for teachers supporting students with ASD. Studies about coaching activities for teachers of elementary and secondary students with ASD are described. The chapter concludes with emerging information on "virtual" or remote coaching delivery methods when face-to-face options are not feasible.

Table 3–1. Training Outcomes Related to Training Components (cf. Joyce & Showers, 2002)

Training Components	Training Outcomes		
	Knowledge of Content	Skill Implementation	Classroom Application
Presentation/ lecture	10%	5%	0%
Plus demonstration	30%	20%	0%
Plus practice	60%	60%	5%
Plus coaching with feedback	95%	95%	95%

Peer-Based Models of Coaching

Peer coaching models emphasize opportunities for teachers, in pairs or in teams, to collaborate and implement new instructional strategies (Joyce & Showers, 1982, 1996). Very often, the process begins with in-service training on an instructional method, followed by shared interaction with a peer or team, and subsequently is followed by an observation in the classroom by one of the peer partners. The process in which teachers go beyond acquiring new instructional methods to full implementation of these techniques is called "transfer." Transfer has to do with mastering an instructional technique so that it easily and flexibly comes under a teacher's "executive control" in the classroom. Executive control enables the individual to think about an approach, "modulate" and "transform it" so that it becomes part of one's teaching repertoire (Joyce & Showers, 1982). The following steps are suggested by Joyce and Showers (1982) to succeed at instructional transfer (Box 3–1).

The first step in transfer is exposure to the theory underlying a new instructional method; the more complex the instructional model, the more intensive is the exposure required to fully comprehend its pedagogical principles—typically, 20 to 30 hours of in-service training is required for this step (Joyce & Showers, 1982). Implementation of an instructional method takes extensive practice and opportunities for exchange with another partner invested in learning

---

Box 3–1. Steps Involved in Transfer of Newly Acquired Instructional Skill(s)

1. Being exposed to the theory underlying the teaching model/method

2. Sharing resources and collaborating with a peer partner to implement the method

3. Planning curriculum and materials with a peer partner

4. Practicing the instructional method in the classroom

5. Demonstrating the instructional method in the classroom with peer observation

6. Reflecting on the impact of the method on student learning

(Based on Joyce & Showers, 1982, 1996.)

the same method (i.e., a peer coach) (Figure 3–1). Peer coaches play an essential role in shared curriculum planning, accessing materials, observation of one another, and reflection on how students are responding. Ultimately, the goal is to successfully adapt a new instructional method to students' needs so that the greatest learning impact is achieved. In a follow-up article, Joyce and Showers (1996) reconceptualized their model of peer coaching and recommend a process of shared observation, coplanning and pooling of resources with, surprisingly, no verbal technical feedback from partners when observing in the classroom. To the extent that verbal feedback becomes evaluative, Joyce and Showers (1996) believe it to be antithetical to the process of collaboration. Instead, these

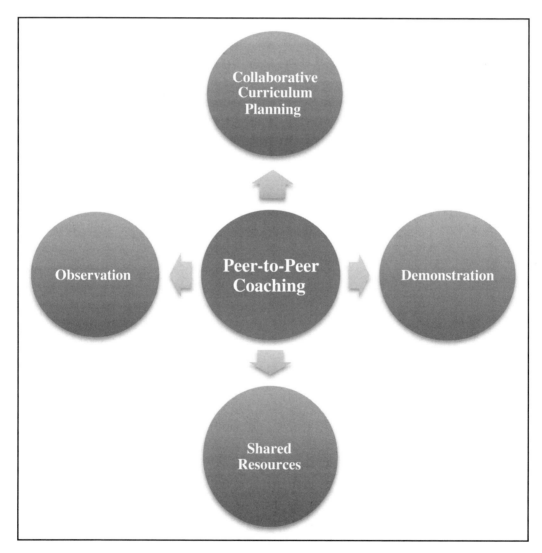

Figure 3–1. Peer-to-peer coaching model (Joyce & Showers, 1996).

authors emphasize a role reversal in peer coaching: the individual teaching is the "coach," while the individual observing becomes the "coached." Observers (i.e., coachees), are present to glean ideas and learn the new instructional practice that they otherwise would not have the benefit of seeing when implementing it on their own. Joyce and Showers (1996) note that coaching entails peers as partners learning from one another and planning collaboratively, reflecting about the impact of their behavior on their students' learning.

Expert Coaching Models

In an alternative approach to peer-based coaching, expert models involve an outside professional, typically someone external to a system with considerable knowledge of an instructional method, who imparts information to a single coachee or an educational team. Allison and Harbour (2009) differentiate coaching and mentoring. In their view, a mentor passes along knowledge and skills, whereas a coach elicits solutions through effective listening and questioning practices. Although recommendations differ in precisely how the coach is engaged in the coaching process, most identify the expert coach as someone with considerable expertise and interpersonal skills. Expert coaching typically involves an initial planning step in which both partners schedule an observation of the classroom and discuss questions or concerns about instructional methods or specific students. Observational visits

are scheduled, and the coach provides technical feedback, either on the same day, or at a later visit. Follow-up meetings can be planned in which coach and coachee clarify information, discuss student outcomes, and address other issues of priority (Figure 3–2). A loop of shared information and goal setting is established between coach and coachee and refined into definable action steps. This feedback loop is essential for developing the coachee's confidence and self-efficacy (Israel, Carnahan, Snyder, & Williamson, 2012).

As we have previously explored in Chapter 1, the relationship of coach and coachee in the expert model should be egalitarian and nonhierarchical. As we examine in vignettes throughout this book, a teacher, or sometimes an administrator, will seek support from the expert by "inviting" the coach into a shared relationship. In this regard, the collaborative aspect of the expert coaching model is similar to peer-based coaching. In a longitudinal study conducted by Becker, Darney, Domitrovich, Pitchford Keperling, and Ialongo (2013), a two-stage expert coaching model was utilized for teachers of general education students in urban schools. In the first stage, teachers received coaching where they were all introduced to a positive behavior prevention program to be implemented daily in classrooms. Coaching sessions followed with opportunities for observation and feedback, modeling, reflection, and data collection by coaches on teacher and student progress with the prevention program. Becker et al. utilized a needs assessment and implemented a second, tailored

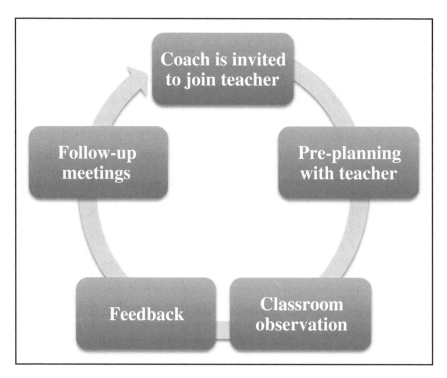

Figure 3–2. Expert coaching model process.

coaching phase personalized to teachers who were slower to progress with classroom implementation of the program. Their customized coaching approach focused on strengthening and reinforcing teacher effectiveness, as well as promoting program sustainability using an assess-plan-do-evaluate strategy. There was system-wide school administrator support for the intervention program implemented through monthly meetings and a framework for classroom walkthrough visits. Although there were many positive outcomes of the tailored coaching method on teacher performance, student behavior, and teacher satisfaction, the authors acknowledged limitations of time constraints of the project's scope and intensity, as well as challenges with program sustainability (Becker et al., 2013).

Cappella, Hamre, Kim, Henry, Frazier, Atkins, and Schoenwald (2012) were interested in what effect different coaching approaches would have with elementary teachers of at-risk students receiving school-based mental health activities in low-income urban schools. The authors assigned classrooms randomly to either a training-only condition, or a teacher training condition supplemented by expert coaching using a behavior intervention program for the classroom. Results indicated that teachers in the training plus coaching condition had a more positive impact on teacher-student interactions for classrooms that originally had low levels of teacher emotional support at the start of the year compared to teachers in the training-only condition. Students in the classrooms with teachers who received training plus coaching also benefited more in terms of their relational closeness to teachers, their social experiences with peers, and their academic self-concept than students in classrooms with teachers in the training-only condition (Cappella et al., 2012).

Other models of instructional coaching have varied the explicit role of coaches from one of technical expert to a "cognitive" coach (Costa & Garmston, 1997). In this model, the coach guides teachers in postinstructional activities as they reflect on their knowledge of instruction through study groups and reading of professional literature on classroom pedagogy (Costa & Garmston, 1997). Cognitive coaches assist educators in consciously reflecting back on their teaching styles and behavior.

Coaching Models for Teachers of Students With ASD

Some of the earliest research on educational coaching was actually conducted with teachers of students with ASD (Koegel, Russo, & Rincover, 1977). Koegel and colleagues (1977) studied the effects of coaching 11 teachers in the use of behavioral instruction techniques derived from the field of applied behavior analysis (ABA) with students with ASD. The teachers were provided with a written manual detailing the instructions for implementing the techniques. They also viewed a video model of the techniques being performed correctly. Next, they attempted to implement the techniques with a student with ASD. Finally,

periodic feedback was provided to the teachers based on their performance implementing the techniques. Results indicated that all 11 teachers rapidly learned to correctly implement the techniques, and that the implementation of these strategies resulted in behavioral gains by the students with ASD (Koegel et al., 1977). These strategies have been used in various combinations across a number of studies, which has resulted in a body of research demonstrating the essential components of successful skill development among teachers and support personnel, referred to as Behavior Skills Training (BST) (Sarokoff & Sturmey, 2004). This multicomponent approach to teaching effective instructional and behavior analytic skills to teachers and support personnel incorporates specific practices that result in transfer of skills from coach to teacher/ support personnel. As seen in Table 3–2, the four research-based components included in BST are instruction, modeling, rehearsal, and feedback (Sarokoff & Sturmey, 2004).

Instruction consists of the coach providing written or verbal information on how to perform a targeted skill/practice, often accompanied with a rationale for why the skill is being taught. Modeling consists of the coach then demonstrating the skill, while the teacher/support personnel observe(s). Rehearsal refers to the teacher performing the skill, often first in a contrived setting, followed by performance of the skill with students in the natural setting. Finally, feedback refers to positive coaching comments in which the coach specifically notes ways in which the skill was performed accurately, along with corrective feedback to

Table 3–2. Components of Behavior Skills Training (BST)

Component	Description
Instruction	Written or verbal information provided describing the skill being taught
Modeling	Demonstration (in person, video-recorded, etc.) of correct use of the skill being taught
Rehearsal	Initial teacher performance of the skill in contrived and/or natural settings
Feedback	Comments from the coach relative to teacher performance of the skill (e.g., praise and error correction)

Note. See Sarokoff and Sturmey (2004).

address any errors made by the teacher/support personnel in demonstrating the skill. Research has demonstrated the effectiveness of the BST package in training teachers to implement a variety of evidence-based practices including discrete trial training (Sarokoff & Sturmey, 2004), paired stimulus preference assessment (Lavie & Sturmey, 2002), mand training (Nigro-Bruzzi & Sturmey, 2010), picture exchange communication systems (PECS) (Homlitas, Rosales, & Candel, 2014; Rosales, Stone, & Rehfeldt, 2009), functional analysis procedures (Ward-Horner & Sturmey, 2012), and naturalistic interventions (Gianoumis, Seiverling & Sturmey, 2012). Furthermore, BST procedures have been used to effectively train teachers in effective practices for addressing a wide range of outcomes for students with ASD, including reducing stereotypy (Dib & Sturmey, 2007), increasing unprompted vocal mands, or requests (Nigro-Bruzzi & Sturmey, 2010), and increasing correct responses during discrete trial training (Sarakoff & Sturmey, 2008). As such, any coaching approach focusing on the transfer of skills to teachers or other personnel, whether it utilizes a peer or expert model, should include the four components of BST within the overall coaching structure and delivery. As subsequent chapters will illustrate, these four components can be utilized in a variety of coaching arrangements, with varying levels of intensity, and to address a variety of effective instructional and behavioral teaching practices for achieving numerous, meaningful outcomes for students with ASD.

Virtual Delivery Methods in Coaching

As literature expands the concept of coaching, educators are discovering multiple means of effectively delivering coaching experiences. The delivery method in the studies mentioned above has focused on face-to-face interaction between coach and coachee. However, recently there has been an examination of remote coaching delivery methods where videoconferencing and other technological equipment make this service available to school districts located in remote settings with special education teachers serving a small population of students with severe disabilities, and/or where access to consultant coaches is not readily available (Harrower & Draper-Rodriguez, 2015). Virtual methods allow greater efficiency for coaches to work with a larger pool of teachers. Israel and colleagues (2012) describe a technology called "virtual bug-in-the-ear" (VBIE), where both novice and experienced teachers receive synchro-nous communication from coaches while instructing students. VBIE technology integrates wireless earpieces and microphones with Internet-based wireless videoconferencing. Coaching is delivered through a teacher's wireless earpiece at intervals throughout the school day (Rock, Gregg, Thead, Acker, Gable, & Zigmond, 2009). Recording of VBIE sessions allows for video review and collaborative reflection by teacher and coach. Israel et al. acknowledge some of the criticisms of this approach, including issues with it being perceived as overly intrusive (i.e., "Big Brother watching") and requiring transparency and oversight to ensure informed consent by teachers and parents, but the benefits of this technology are prom-

---

Box 3–2. Benefits of Virtual Bug-in-the-Ear Coaching

■ Supporting teachers in providing adequate student response time

■ Helping manage immediate behavior situations

■ Scaffolding effective communication techniques with students

■ Planning and implementing instructional strategies, accommodations, and adaptations

■ Modeling and coaching specific instructional strategies for the teacher

■ Providing program monitoring of student learning outcomes

■ Problem solving alternative assessments and assessment methods

(Based on Israel, Carnahan, Snyder, & Williamson, 2012.)

ising (see Box 3–2). When embedded with supportive activities, such as collaborative reflection between coach and coachee and ongoing professional development, virtual coaching has been found to result in comparable outcomes to those found in face-to-face coaching (Rock et al., 2009; Ruble et al., 2013).

In a virtual coaching study, Machalicek and colleagues (2010) examined how well six teachers implemented functional analysis procedures to assess challenging behaviors in children with ASD while they received performance feedback in a video teleconferencing format. This feedback was provided from a university supervisor who had prerecorded classroom sessions using an Internet-based video Web camera. Results indicated that all six teachers were successful in maintaining what they had learned 5 weeks after training, although there was a decline in their skill retention thereafter (Machalicek et al., 2010).

Summary

A variety of different models and delivery methods for educational coaching have been proposed and evaluated for supporting teachers. Most approaches can be categorized as either peer-based or expert coaching. Peer coaching models involve teacher dyads, or teams, that have a shared investment in learning a new instructional method or pedagogy, whereas expert coaching models involve ongoing embedded support of a teacher, or coachee, by someone with both interpersonal skills and instructional exper-

tise. Both coaching models have been shown to be effective in altering teacher skills and perceptions, enhancing learning outcomes for parent/caregivers and students, as well as improving behavior for students with ASD.

Significant and positive learning effects also hold for face-to-face and virtual coaching delivery methods. Virtual coaching made readily available through expanding technological resources is an efficient way to support teachers and school districts in remote or isolated settings. Regardless of the advantages of technological versus face-to-face coaching approaches, there are striking similarities in the essential components and activities that coaches use to establish collaboration and embed supportive practices with those they coach. These include shared family and teacher priorities for student support, collaborative problem solving to establish instructional or IEP objectives, reflective questioning, demonstration and/or modeling of instructional techniques, and ongoing professional development for the teacher. Although controlled studies evaluating the sustainability of instructional learning by teachers indicate a need for intensive coaching, emerging research has underscored the benefit of coaching to improve the quality of IEPs and for teacher and family satisfaction (Kucharczyk et al, 2012; Woods, Wilcox, Friedman, & Murch, 2011). Regardless of the coaching model (e.g., peer-based, expert-based, etc.) or delivery method (e.g., face to face, virtual, etc.), the four evidence-based practices of instruction, modeling, rehearsal, and feedback as encapsulated in Behavior Skills Training (Sarokoff & Sturmey, 2004) should be embedded when the goal is to build new skills for the individual being coached. Up to this point, guidance on the selection of the coaching model and the coaching delivery method for specific support needs of teachers of students with ASD has not been provided. The next chapter will introduce such a framework, with subsequent chapters illustrating how to implement effective coaching supports across a variety of coaching methods and targeting essential skills needed by teachers to effectively support students with ASD.

End-of-Chapter Questions

1. Compare peer and expert coaching models. What elements are shared by these approaches? What are their differences?

2. Assume you are a special education administrator at a school and are tasked with ensuring that a novice teacher servicing a classroom of students with ASD is provided with quality teacher induction. Make a case for electing to go with either a peer-based or an expert coaching model. How would you justify the expense of using one or the other coaching approach with your Board of Education?

3. You are coaching a new teacher to learn how to use an evidence-based practice for students with ASD. Select a skill to teach and develop a plan for using the four compo-

nents of Behavior Skills Training (BST) (see Table 3–2) to teach this skill. Be sure to provide examples for how you will address each of the four components.

4. What is the difference between face-to-face and virtual methods of coaching? When would you use one or the other approach?

References

Allison, S. & Harbour, M. (2009). The coaching toolkit. *British Journal of Educational Technology, 40*(6), 1142.

Becker, K. D., Darney, D., Domitrovich, C., Pitchford Keperling, J., & Ialongo, N. S. (2013). Supporting universal prevention programs: A two-phased coaching model. *Clinical Child and Family Psychology Review, 16*(2), 213–228.

Cappella, E., Hamre, B. K., Kim, H. Y., Henry, D. B., Frazier, S., Atkins, M. & Schoenwald, S. K. (2012). Teacher consultation and coaching within mental health practice: Classroom and child effects in urban elementary schools. *Journal Consulting and Clinical Psychology, 80*(4), 597–610.

Costa, A., & Garmston, R. (1997). *Cognitive coaching: A foundation for renaissance schools* (3rd ed.). Norwood, MA: Christopher-Gordon.

Denton, C. A., & Hasbrouck, J. (2009). A description of instructional coaching and its relationship to consultation. *Journal of Educational & Psychological Consultation, 19,* 150–175.

Dib, N., & Sturmey, P. (2007). Reducing student stereotypy by improving teachers' implementation of discrete-trial teaching. *Journal of Applied Behavior Analysis, 40*(2), 339–343.

Gianoumis, S., Seiverling, L., & Sturmey, P. (2012), The effects of behavior skills training on correct teacher implementation of natural language paradigm teaching skills and child behavior. *Behavioral Intervention, 27,* 57–74

Hanft, B. E., Rush, D. D., & Shelden, M. L. (2004). *Coaching families and colleagues in early childhood.* Baltimore, MD: Brookes.

Harrower, J. K., & Draper-Rodriguez, C. (2015). Using mobile technology for student teaching observations of special education candidates. In S. Keengwe (Ed.), *Advancing higher education with mobile learning technologies: Cases, trends and inquiry-based methods.* Hershey, PA: IGI Global.

Homlitas, C., Rosales, R., & Candel, L. (2014). A further evaluation of behavior skills training for implementation of the picture exchange communication system. *Journal of Applied Behavior Analysis, 47*(1), 1–6.

Israel, M., Carnahan C. R., Snyder, K. K., & Williamson, P. (2012). Supporting new teachers of students with significant disabilities through virtual coaching: A proposed model. *Remedial and Special Education, 34*(4), 195–204.

Joyce, B., & Showers, B. (1982). The coaching of teaching. *Educational Leadership, 40*(1), 4–10.

Joyce, B., & Showers, B. (1996). The evolution of peer coaching. *Educational Leadership, 53*(6), 12–16.

Joyce, B., & Showers, B. (2002). *Student achievement through staff development* (3rd ed.). Alexandria, VA: Association for Supervision and Curriculum.

Koegel, R. L., Russo, D. C., & Rincover, A. (1977). Assessing and training teachers in the generalized use of behavior modification with autistic children. *Journal of Applied Behavior Analysis, 10,* 197–205.

Kucharczyk, S., Shaw, E., Smith Myles, B., Sullivan, L., Szidon, K., & Tuchman-Ginsberg, L. (2012). *Guidance and coaching on evidence-based practices for learners with autism spectrum disorders.* Chapel Hill, NC: University of North Carolina, Frank Porter Graham Child Development Institute, National Professional Development Center on Autism Spectrum Disorders.

Lavie, T., & Sturmey, P. (2002). Training staff to conduct a paired-stimulus preference assessment. *Journal of Applied Behavior Analysis, 35,* 209–211.

Malchalicek, W., Rispoli, M., Lang, R., O'Reilly, M. F., Davis, T., & Hetlinger Franco, J. (2010). Training teachers to assess challenging behaviors of students with autism using video teleconferencing. *Education & Training in Autism and Developmental Disabilities, 45*(2), 203–215.

Nigro-Bruzzi, D., & Sturmey, P. (2010). The effects of behavioral skills training on mand training by staff and unprompted vocal mands by children. *Journal of Applied Behavior Analysis, 43*(4), 757–761.

Rock, M. L., Gregg, M., Thead, B. K., Acker, S. E., Gable, R. A., & Zigmond, N. P. (2009). Can you hear me now? Evaluation of an online wireless technology to provide real-time feedback to special education teachers in training. *Teacher Education and Special Education, 32,* 64–82.

Rosales, R., Stone, K., & Rehfeldt, R. A. (2009). The effects of a behavioral skills training on implementation of the picture exchange communication system. *Journal of Applied Behavior Analysis, 42,* 541–549.

Ruble, L., McGrew, J. H., Toland, M. D., Dalrymple, N. J., & Jung, L. A. (2013). A randomized controlled trial of COMPASS Web-based and face-to-face teacher coaching in autism. *Journal of Consulting and Clinical Psychology, 81*(3), 566–572.

Sarokoff, R. A., & Sturmey, P. (2004). The effects of behavioral skills training on staff implementation of discrete-trial teaching. *Journal of Applied Behavior Analysis, 37*(4), 535–538.

Sarokoff, R. A., & Sturmey, P. (2008). The effects of instructions, rehearsal, modeling, and feedback on acquisition and generalization of staff use of discrete trial teaching and student correct responses. *Research in Autism Spectrum Disorders, 2*(1), 125–136.

Ward-Horner, J., & Sturmey, P. (2012). Component analysis of behavior skills training in functional analysis. *Behavioral Interventions, 27,* 75–92.

Woods, J. J., & Maturana, E. (2010). *From a distance: Using performance-based video feedback for mentoring.* Chapel Hill, NC: National Early Childhood Technical Assistance Center.

Woods, J. J., Wilcox, J. J., Friedman, M., & Murch, T. (2011). Collaborative consultation in natural environments: Strategies to enhance family-centered supports and services. *Language, Speech, and Hearing Services in Schools, 42,* 379–392.

CHAPTER 4

Key Attributes of Effective Coaching

Seek opportunities to show you care. The smallest gestures often make the biggest difference.
—John Wooden

Chapter Objectives

- Examine key communication styles that promote positive interactions between a coach and educators working with students with autism spectrum disorder (ASD)

- Establish a coach-coachee relationship to ensure mutual trust, confidence, credibility, and shared commitment

- Establish a coachee's commitment to change

- Understand the power of a positive/growth mindset

- Learn how to develop an action plan/vision with preliminary milestones and timelines

- Use solution-finding techniques

- Explore how to strive for mastery

Introduction

High-quality coaching relies on being able to communicate effectively. In any coaching situation, the coach must listen closely to what is being said, both verbally and nonverbally, acknowledge feelings, and if the situation calls for it, articulate a plan of action. Sometimes just listening to another person opens up options that the individual could not visualize or understand. Communication is the heart and soul of coaching. If any change is going to be made, either in skill development, behavior, or both, it must start with openness and trust, the cornerstones of honest interpersonal relationships (Box 4–1).

Establishing Collaborative Relationships Between the Coach and Teacher

Coach and teacher must treat each other with equal respect and in a consistent manner. By establishing this type of collaborative relationship, both parties mutually contribute to the success of the affiliation. A collaborative relationship involves four critical elements:

1. Two parties **reciprocally communicate** with one another where the interchange is based on trust and respect.

2. Team members work to **find solutions** to pressing problems.

3. Both parties make a **commitment to execute a plan of action**.

4. Both **strive toward mastery** of items/factors identified in a plan of action.

In a collaborative relationship, there is an agreement between two parties that an action or change will take place. In many ways the action plan becomes a mutually agreed upon contract where both parties cooperate together and control the decision making. Without these four critical elements of a collaborative relationship between a coach and teacher, little behavior change and/or new skill acquisition by the teaching staff and students will take place. It must be noted that change in adult behavior usually occurs when an adult becomes aware of his or her behavior patterns and/or attitudes, practices different ways of responding, applies the changes across settings, and then receives ongoing support. By establishing a collaborative relationship, a coach can provide support through this change process for new learning to occur without the learner feeling intimidated or overwhelmed. Collaborative learning, which entails sharing one's experiences, communicating responsibly, and working together to arrive at solutions is a highly effective way to obtain and impart knowledge and skills. Collaboration offers an immediate way for coach and coachee to establish a positive and professional relationship.

Reciprocal Communication

As indicated, reciprocal communication between two individuals relies on trust and shared respect. A few key concepts undergird reciprocal communication.

Box 4–1. Vignette: Who Is the Teacher Here?

My name is Pricilla Newcomer, and I have just started my first assignment as a special educator in a class with seven upper elementary students with ASD. Five of the students have a one-to-one behavioral aide funded by the school district, and the other two students are high functioning on the autism spectrum and included in general education classes for most of the day with support from my instructional assistant. Since I am a new teacher, I am struggling with assessing where my kids are at both socially and academically. The one-to-one aides use a system provided by an outside agency to gather detailed data designed to help improve behavior and social communication, but which is rarely reviewed. Though I am grateful for their assistance, I am having a great deal of trouble assessing my students in reference to the state standards and their IEP goals. Although their IEP goals are written to improve social communication and basic academics, for the five with one-to-one services, the reality is that the aides directly control the students' social interactions. We provide very few naturalistic opportunities for students to spontaneously interact with each other and the world around them. Everything in my class for those five students is controlled, and I feel that I have little say in what goes on in *my* classroom. I wonder each day, "Who is the teacher here?"

One of my strengths is good old "kid watching" and using what I see to develop a program to meet their needs. I am also part of the general education team meetings for my included students. I am increasing my knowledge and understanding of the state standards (Common Core) and how to incorporate grade-level assessment into my program along with meeting students' IEP goals. I have excellent rapport with my instructional assistant and the general education teachers. Our meetings together have focused on appropriate student assessment. I feel that this peer-to-peer interaction has been helpful to all of us. Unfortunately, I am not able to communicate what I think should be accomplished in the classroom with the one-on-one aides because of the influence of the outside agency and their approach to copious data collection with little subsequent analysis. I need help from an outside consultant.

They include maintaining a positive mindset when interacting with others, knowing that the way you say something is more important than what is being said (content versus delivery), and listening attentively when a person speaks. Classrooms where educators work with students with ASD are dynamic environments, and ongoing communication is standard operating procedure. Knowing how to communicate effectively and efficiently cements collaborative relationships. Idol, Paoloucci-Whitcomb & Nevin (2000) and Knight (2007) emphasize the importance of "egalitarian" and "nonhierarchical" relationships between coach and coachee as key attributes of reciprocal communication (see Chapter 1).

Positive Mindset

Carol Dweck, Stanford University professor and developer of the "growth mindset" concept defines a mindset as a "fixed mental attitude or disposition that predetermines a person's responses to and interpretations of situations," or a growth mindset, where people believe that their most basic abilities can be developed through dedication and hard work. Intellect and talent are just the starting point. This view creates a love of learning and a resilience that is essential for great accomplishment (Dweck, 2007). Staying open to new ideas, maintaining a flexible attitude, and remaining positive and resilient are "growth mindset" qualities essential to working with and teaching students with ASD. An educator with a growth mindset impacts students and staff alike

and sets the tone of the classroom. A collaborative relationship calls for all individuals working with students to develop and maintain a positive mindset, especially when the students and the learning environment present unexpected challenges. Flare-ups occur frequently in individuals with ASD requiring educators to anticipate needs and preempt challenging behavior before matters escalate. Without a doubt, student behavior and learning problems can also lead to tension between adults. Oftentimes coaches are asked to consult in classrooms where the adults have significant trouble getting along with one another, and the work atmosphere is strained. A coach can identify these "hot spots" as evidenced in the vignette *Buyer's Remorse* (see Chapter 1, Box 1–5) where a teacher struggles with negative interpersonal interactions with too many adults in the classroom. Negative interchanges between adults invariably leads to hurt feelings, poor or improper decisions, and increased classroom tension. Coaches can help educators act positively toward one another, rather than act or react negatively. In these situations, the coach observes adult interaction in the classroom, identifies areas where communication between two adults appears tense, debriefs with the affected parties at an arranged time to discuss what was observed (***reciprocal communication***), and then develops an action plan to preempt or counteract communication difficulties (***execute a plan of action***). By remaining positive and objective, the coach deescalates conflict or potential conflict. Through attentive listening, nonjudgmental responding, and clear, direct, and open communication, the coach preserves the integrity of the relationship(s), offering constructive solutions and action-oriented steps that can be reviewed and worked on over time (***strive toward mastery/sustainability***).

A positive learning environment allows students to feel safe and non-threatened. It also has a calming effect, so important when establishing classroom routines. Communication is much like a boomerang: what goes around comes around. Motivational speaker Zig Ziglar maintains that "positive thinking will let you do everything better than negative thinking will." Coaches who act positively have a distinct advantage in that adults in the classroom will generally respond positively, and this, in turn, carries over to other adult interactions. Coaches who adopt a positive mindset not only support adults working with students with ASD to develop appropriate ways of dealing with challenges, but also offset a teacher's fixed mindset that sometimes emerges with misperceptions or ingrained attitudes (e.g., "Kids with ASD just behave that way"; "General education teachers don't understand"; "Some parents think they know better than the teacher").

Delivery Versus Content

Along with a positive mindset, another key component of establishing collaborative relationships centers on the message delivery (how things are said), rather than the content (what is said). The adage, "It's not what you say; it's how you say it," underpins most communication and is a central feature of collaborative relationships. Many interpersonal problems arise from the way people communicate, both verbally and nonverbally. The way things are said, along with accompanying body language, can lead to misunderstanding and mistrust. The vignette in Box 4–2 highlights how one's demeanor can lead to problems in communication.

Once again, it's all about the delivery, and not so much about what was said, or the content of the message. In the second situation in this vignette, the assistant feels valued and appreciated and given an opportunity to make a decision to support instruction for Jesse, rather than feeling obligated to do an activity that may be contrary to what he or she knows works best for the student. Obviously, there is no excuse for the way the assistant initially communicated, and that still needs to be dealt with along with, for that matter, the way the teacher responded. A coach would suggest alternative ways to handle interpersonal conflict, pointing out the benefit of making comments in a proactive manner. Role-playing scenarios, such as the one provided in the vignette in Box 4–2, prove helpful in gaining an understanding of how communication influences behavior and vice versa. In reciprocal communication both parties strive to understand one another and take responsibility for awkward interchanges by acknowledging their mistakes and determining how best to interact with one another. In this example, a coach must remain neutral with the intent of helping both parties gain an enhanced

Box 4–2. Vignette: Pushing My Buttons

An instructional assistant says in a surly voice when asked to work with a small group of students with ASD on a writing activity, "I don't think that we should do that; it's way over their heads and Jesse will just flip out. Plus, we've never done it before." A teacher's immediate response might be one of restrained anger, punctuated by a stern tone and facial expression: "Please just do it. I know that this is exactly what Jesse needs." The assistant might defer with a reluctant, "Okay," as if to communicate: "It won't work, but I'll do it anyway." Notice how this interaction leads to more communication problems between the teacher and assistant. Both parties now have to figure out a way to resolve their differences, which may or not happen that day or the next. The delay often reinforces differences of opinions, which makes resolution more difficult. Even when the parties do come together they may not address their core communication problems, and the teacher may gloss over it with a cursory "I'm sorry about the way I talked with you the other day." The assistant may or may not accept the apology, or shrug it off.

Now let's see how the teacher and assistant might have handled the same situation in a more constructive and appropriate manner in the following role-play.

Teacher: "You know I was thinking the same thing and appreciate that you know what sets Jesse off. Let's give it a go and be ready to allow Jesse to go to his 'cooldown' strategy if he can't handle it. Thanks."

Instructional Assistant: "No problem. Jesse needs to be challenged academically. I'd like to see if he could actually do it. Cooldown is a good backup plan for him."

understanding of how they communicate so that instruction for students is not compromised (***reciprocal communication***). The coach asks both parties if communicating in this fashion helps or hinders their relationship, and then invites them to discuss their thoughts. The coach may jot down a few of their thoughts and then summarizes the conversation. If needed, the coach continues the discussion to ensure closure. Next the coach with the teacher and instructional assistant develop an action plan (***execute a plan of action***) with clear steps for improvement in their communication concentrating on how things are said to one another (**delivery versus content**). The action plan would have a timeline for the coach to follow up with both parties at prescribed intervals until improvement in interpersonal communication is noticeable. In situations where a communication breakdown occurs, an action plan is key to sustaining change in behavior. Requesting signatures when both parties have completed the action plan steps often creates a sense of ownership for the change (***strive toward mastery/sustainability***).

Attentive Listening

Expert coaches listen attentively to what others have to say, and then paraphrase or summarize what was said. Some suggested replies are, "Thanks for sharing. Let me see if I understand what you said"; "That's an interesting way to look at that. I hadn't thought of that in that way"; "Could you tell me more?" Responses that are honest and show genuine interest garner trust and respect between coach and coachee and other parties. Attentive listening is the cornerstone of communication in collaborative relationships. It is incumbent upon the coach, teaching staff, and other stakeholders to make a concerted effort to listen to one another and clarify any communication that could lead to a

potential misunderstanding. This is also true for communication between and among other adults in the classroom.

In another case, an outside consultant working with a behavior agency contracted by the school district visits a teacher's classroom once a week for 2 hours. During that time the consultant gives the teacher instruction, interacts with students in an overly firm manner, and basically disrupts the classroom routine. The visit creates undue and unnecessary tension between the teacher and the consultant, and when the teacher offers a thought or suggestion, the consultant dismisses it. The student, who is prone to outbursts when routines are disrupted, reacts to the situation, biting his hand, increasing the tension between teacher and consultant as well as others in the classroom. Although unexpected, conflicting situations like these can happen in settings where students with ASD are served.

Coaches may be called in to mediate uncomfortable interactions. In the above scenario, it is imperative that the coach maintains a positive mindset when interacting with the teacher and the outside consultant. As the coach enters this classroom, the teacher might corner the coach and say in a taciturn manner that the consultant is "negative, doesn't listen, and is a know-it-all." The first goal regarding this interaction is to seek clarification. By listening to and acknowledging the teacher's feelings and gaining an understanding of the situation, the coach can help the teacher identify a means to communicate responsibly and professionally with the consultant. The coach may also talk to the consultant to ascertain his or her part of the situation. Listening to each person's side of the story to make sure that a positive result occurs between both parties makes it more likely that the student will be consistently taught or followed up with in an appropriate manner. Discerning those areas where both parties can come to understand one another requires skill and patience from a coach. Sometimes people just rub each other the wrong way, and the coach, after listening attentively, can advise an appropriate action.

Solution-Finding Process

Too often problems arise in classrooms without a solution in sight. The problem may seem incidental to an outside observer, or for that matter, even a skilled coach called in to help. However, communication is always about the small stuff—the less than obvious verbal and nonverbal communication between people that left unattended festers into frustration and conflict. Finding a solution without a roadmap to do so usually means that an undercurrent of communication problems continues to exist until an individual either blows up, or gives up. To offset potential communication flare-ups, the following 10-step solution-finding process has proven helpful to building the coach and coachee relationship (Table 4–1). When working toward a solution, it is always helpful to have materials to visualize your progress toward reaching your goal (e.g., chart paper and markers).

Execute a Plan of Action

Learning how to communicate effectively encourages positive collaborative relationships. Ongoing communication acts as the glue to execute a plan of action ensuring that skills are learned and carried out in a clear and direct manner with and for students. Teaching requires sophisticated reciprocal communication with all stakeholders who interact with students in and out of the classroom. That being said, an essential function of a coach's role is to increase the skill set of the teacher or educational team in a specific teaching/learning environment. Once both the coach and teacher know how to communicate reciprocally, have and maintain a positive mindset, and attentively listen to one another, there can be a focus on applying new instructional strategies, which may elicit further problem solving. As a case in point, a teacher explains to the coach that one of her high school students lacks motivation in testing situations. She knows that the student has the ability to pass the high school exit exam but appears unmotivated. The coach in this situation knows the student fairly well, and after discussing the matter with the teacher, both decide that the student does not understand the relevance or importance of trying to do his or best on the test. They both agree to devise an action plan using a Classroom Action Plan form (Table 4–2) to identify goals and implementation steps. Using the Classroom Action Plan form gives the coach and teacher objective steps to make changes to help the student achieve test-taking success. Motivation

Table 4–1. Solution-Finding Worksheet

1. Identify a few goals	
2. Brainstorm ideas	
3. Prioritize immediate goal	
4. Organize materials	
5. Discuss and jot down barriers	
6. Clarify goals	
7. Develop an action plan	
8. Develop a follow-up plan	
9. Evaluate progress	
10. Celebrate success	

Table 4–2. Classroom Action Plan Form

Student Name: Tom

Short-term objective: To improve test-taking skills

Barriers: Lack of motivation—gives up easily, fidgety, quits in middle of test

Program objective: To provide multiple opportunities for capable students to pass the high school exit exam

Implementation Steps	Responsibilities *Who will do it?*	Resources *People, materials*	Time *Day/Month*
Practice tests with reduced number of items	Tom	Teacher or Instructional Assistant (IA); Teacher-constructed tests	Mornings
Timer for test completion with a reward (computer game)	Teacher, IA	Auditory or visual timer, preferred computer game	Monday and Wednesday during independent time
Identify specific times for encouragement and make the encouragement meaningful (e.g., "Way to stay focused, Tom, you're beating the timer")	Teacher or IA	Auditory or visual timer set at timed intervals	Mondays (M),Wednesdays (W) during independent time
Keep data on how many practice items Tom completes	Teacher, IA	Data-keeping forms	M, W Independent time
Increase number of items on the test	Tom	Teacher, IA; Teacher-constructed test items	M,W Independent time
Take practice tests twice a week	Tom	Teacher, IA	

can be tricky with high school students in general, and even more so with adolescents with ASD. An action plan provides the foundation for collecting data important for monitoring student progress and making program adjustments.

Table 4–2 outlines how the coach and teacher decided to tackle this student's test-taking motivation using the Classroom Action Plan form.

The critical skills of identifying a problem, developing actionable steps to solve the problem, collecting and analyzing data relevant to the problem, debriefing by the coach with staff, and adjusting or changing an instructional approach based on that data emanate from a well-thought-out action plan. Taking into consideration the demands on the instructional team, a coach can offer suggestions, model the skill if need be, and provide tangible resources; for example, assistive technology supports, social scripts, or visual supports. Once the action plan has been initiated, a follow-up plan is helpful as well. By having an action plan, the coach and teacher can immediately review progress and make modifications to it.

Not all coach and teacher interactions require an action plan. For example, suggesting alternative room arrangements for enhanced classroom mobility, or different seating arrangements are actionable steps that are clearly achieved by immediate implementation by coach and teacher. Nevertheless, learning to arrange a room and seating to maximize student learning is definitely an early skill that requires some degree of coaching support for new teachers. In these kinds of activities, the coach may include additional classroom staff and educational team members so that they can also provide input to suggested changes or alternative arrangements.

Striving for Mastery and Sustainability

Learning a new skill and then implementing it for the first time can be an exhilarating experience for a teacher. Putting that skill into practice on a reg-

ular basis, however, is a challenge for both novice and experienced teachers. To strive for skill mastery, the coachee must be open to ongoing processes of learning and experience. Educational coaching experts refer to these intrapersonal growth processes as "reflection" and "self-efficacy" (Rush, Shelden & Raab, 2008; Sheridan, Welch, & Orme, 1996), which ultimately shore up teacher personal satisfaction and self-confidence. Receiving authentic and consistent feedback from a coach, and then implementing suggestions increases teacher skill acquisition. Consistency in application of a new instructional strategy or skill, in turn, yields positive outcomes for students with a diagnosis of ASD. The scope and comprehensiveness of strategies needed to effectively instruct students with this disability are best learned through practice with guidance and embedded support from a coach, rather than through trial-and-error implementation. In several coaching studies, systematic "performance feedback" to special education teachers has been successfully documented for promoting children's social competence in early childhood programs (Fox, Hemmeter, Snyder, Perez-Binder, & Clarke, 2011), coaching parents of young children with social communication and language delays (Woods, Wilcox, Friedman, & Murch, 2011) and parents of young children with ASD (Kucharczyk, Shaw, Smith-Myles, Sullivan, Szidon, & Tuchman-Ginsberg, 2012). As mentioned previously in Chapter 3, the use of video technology and virtual coaching methods achieves these same positive outcomes as does face-to-face coaching methods with special educators (Ruble, Birdwhistell, Toland, & McGrew, 2011; Ruble, McGrew, Toland, Dalrymple, & Jung, 2014). Regardless of the coaching delivery model utilized, effective coaches consistently demonstrate and provide a common set of key attributes, as highlighted in Table 4–3.

As previously reviewed, learning a new teaching skill, practicing it over time, and receiving support and acknowledgement from a coach or mentor ensures that the skill will be learned and sustained over time. Educators refer to that degree of mastery of a skill or strategy as having it in their "tool belt," which means a teacher knows the skill or strategy so well that it can be used when needed. In essence, an educator has mastered it much like a skilled gymnast has mastered a movement routine. Although new competencies may not be as well practiced as routine competencies, mastering new skills to teach students with ASD is important given the unique strengths and needs of this population of students. Getting comfort-

able using a new skill, receiving the necessary support from a mentor or coach, and then implementing the skill consistently lead to mastery.

Summary

High-quality coaching aims to increase the awareness and responsibility of both the teacher and the coach. Key attributes of a positive mindset and attentive listening enhance reciprocal communication between parties when there is conflict. These attributes enable progression to problem solving solutions with an action plan and commitment to skill mastery. Under the direction of a high-quality and expert coach, teachers learn how to develop and maintain a positive collaborative relationship through effective communication, develop and master skills, and learn how to deliver instruction in a robust fashion, so that students with ASD receive the most productive education possible.

Table 4–3. Key Attributes of Effective Coaching

- Collaboration
- Reciprocal communication
- Joint goal planning
- Self-reflection
- Problem solving
- Performance feedback
- Ongoing professional development support

End-of-Chapter Questions

1. How do you think your coworkers see you? Think about this question prior to answering it. Please write a complete paragraph or two, or write a series of bullet points articulating your response clearly.

2. After reading the vignette in Box 4–1, "Who Is the Teacher Here?," jot down a few of the key points that resonate for you. The teacher is pleading for

help from an outside consultant or coach to help her sort through the situation at hand. How do you think a coach can help her resolve some of her feelings?

3. As stated, communication is like a boomerang: What goes around comes around. Working with students with ASD requires thoughtful communication. Describe a time when your communication was less than thoughtful and was based on a fixed mindset rather than a growth mindset. What happened, and how did you finally resolve the issue? This can be a personal issue, or related to the classroom in which you teach.

4. In the situation described in the vignette "Pushing My Buttons," find a colleague and role-play this interaction as spelled out in the vignette. After doing so, discuss how you would have handled this situation differently. Make sure to talk about the content of the message versus the way in which something is said. Now analyze the way you say things with other professionals or with others in general, and jot down two or three ways you can improve your delivery in challenging and nonchallenging situations.

5. Form a triad, and have one person in the triad assume the role of "the coach" using the "Pushing My Buttons" vignette presented in Box 4–2 as your prompt, and coach both parties in understanding that how you say something can create or relieve tension. Change roles so everyone role-plays the coach's role. The coach can start the conversation with this prompt: "It's good that we have an opportunity to discuss what happened this morning. I am very pleased that you both resolved the situation amicably, but I want to make sure that we continue to communicate responsibly. Let me start by indicating it's not what you say, it's how you say it that can cause problems in relationships. Each member of the triad should finish the role-play accenting his or her individual style of interaction.

6. In classrooms where students with ASD are served, educators have a tendency to manage the problem rather than solve the problem. Using the Solution-Finding Steps/Plan (see Table 4–1), identify an issue/problem that needs to be solved. If you are not currently a teacher or educator working with students with ASD or other special needs, identify an area in your life that needs to be solved and use the Solution-Finding Steps/Plan to make the goal attainable.

7. Review the Classroom Action Plan Form (see Table 4–2) written for the high school student with high-functioning ASD, who is unmotivated to pass the high school exam. Identify a student and a specific behavior you want to address, and develop a classroom action plan for that student. Use the Classroom Action Plan Form and clearly identify the implementation steps, responsibilities, resources, and time frame to accomplish the steps.

References

Dweck, C. (2007). *Mindset: The new psychology of success.* New York, NY: Random House.

Fox, L., Hemmeter, M. L., Snyder, P., Perez Binder, D., & Clarke, S. (2011). Coaching early childhood special educators to implement a comprehensive model for promoting young children's social competence. *Topics in Early Childhood Special Education, 31,* 178–191.

Idol, L., Paoloucci-Whitcomb, P., & Nevin, A. (2000). *Collaborative consultation.* Austin, TX: Pro-Ed.

Israel, M., Carnahan, C. R., Snyder, K. K., & Williamson, P. (2012). Supporting new teachers of students with significant disabilities through virtual coaching: A proposed model. *Remedial and Special Education, 34*(4), 195–204.

Knight, J. (2007). *Instructional coaching: A partnership approach to improving instruction.* Thousand Oaks, CA: Corwin Press.

Kucharczyk, S., Shaw, E., Smith Myles, B., Sullivan, L., Szidon, K., & Tuchman-Ginsberg, L. (2012). *Guidance and coaching on evidence-based practices for learners with autism spectrum disorders.* Chapel Hill, NC: University of North Carolina, Frank Porter Graham Child Development Institute, National Professional Development Center on Autism Spectrum Disorders.

Ruble, L., Birdwhistell, J., Toland, M. D., & McGrew, J. H. (2011). Analysis of parent, teacher, and consultant speech exchanges and educational outcomes of students with autism during COMPASS consultation. *Journal of Educational and Psychological Consultation, 21*(4), 259–283.

Ruble, L., McGrew, J. H., Toland, M. D., Dalrymple, N. J., & Jung, L. A. (2014). A randomized controlled trial of COMPASS Web-based and face-to-face teacher coaching in autism. *Journal of Consulting and Clinical Psychology, 81*(3), 566–572.

Rush, D. D., Shelden, M. L., & Raab, M. (2008). A framework for reflective questioning when using a coaching interaction style. *CASEtools: Instruments and Procedures for Implementing Early Childhood and Family Support Practices, 4*(1), 1–7.

Sheridan, S. M., Welch, M., & Orme, S. F. (1996). Is consultation effective? A review of outcome research. *Remedial and Special Education, 17*(6), 341–354.

Woods, J. J., Wilcox, J. J., Friedman, M., & Murch, T. (2011). Collaborative consultation in natural environments: Strategies to enhance family-centered supports and services. *Language, Speech and Hearing Services in Schools, 42,* 379–392.

CHAPTER 5

High-Quality Coaching: A Framework

The ability to help the people around me self-actualize their goals underlines the single aspect of my abilities and the label that I value most—teacher.

—Bill Walsh

Chapter Objectives

■ Overview a multitiered framework for coaching on the basis of a three-tiered model of support

■ Assist teachers and districts in identifying the type of coaching supports needed for successful implementation of instructional and behavioral interventions for students with autism spectrum disorder (ASD)

■ Prioritize coaching goals and coaching strategies for three levels of coaching intensity

■ Offer coaching strategies for establishing collaborative working relationships

---

Introduction

Coaching is not something you get. It is something you do with others to earn their trust and respect with the potential to change lives for the better. Traditional models of coaching emphasize an expert imparting knowledge to a novice learner, demonstrating a skill or way of doing that maximizes the potential of the learner, group, or team. The expert provides an invaluable service, if and only if he or she can communicate with the new learner(s), monitor growth, and evaluate progress. High-quality coaching (HQC) embraces and accentuates equality in the coach-coachee relationship as well as empowerment for the coachee (see Cramer, 1998; Kampwirth & Powers, 2011). Face-to-face coaching stresses the principle of live coaching, where a coach with knowledge of evidence-based practices shares a strategy that a teacher or educational team may find useful with a particular student, or demonstrates how to target a particular challenging behavior of a student. The teacher, likewise, can demonstrate that instructional method to an instructional assistant for use with an individual student. Oftentimes, instructional assistants, many of whom have been with a classroom for years, have acquired strategies that the teacher or coach may find incredibly practical. High-quality coaching provides opportunities for all stakeholders in the classroom to share ideas that build camaraderie, trust, and newfound skills. The following coaching approaches can be used independently, or in some combination depending on the particular teaching circumstance.

In Chapter 1, we emphasized the trend toward mentoring professional staff that teach students with special needs and, in particular, those with ASD. Coaching efforts require attention to the elements that make it exceptional and worthwhile. In this chapter, we clarify a framework for coaching delineating how this process can be undertaken at different levels of intensity. Borrowing from multitiered systems of support and decision-making logic utilized by an increasing number of fields of educational methods (e.g., response to intervention, positive behavior interventions and supports, etc.), we conceptualize three levels of coaching intensity that can be used to make system-wide decisions about the allocation of coaching resources and activities by a given educational agency (e.g., county office of education, local education agency or school district, public school consortium, etc.). Each level of coaching intensity is selected on the basis of need and context within a given school program or classroom (Figure 5–1).

Intensity of Coaching

All teachers can benefit from a basic level of coaching support by accessing peers and/or educational professionals knowledgeable about special needs students to serve as a support system, and thus, our first level of coaching is referred to as "peer-to-peer coaching."

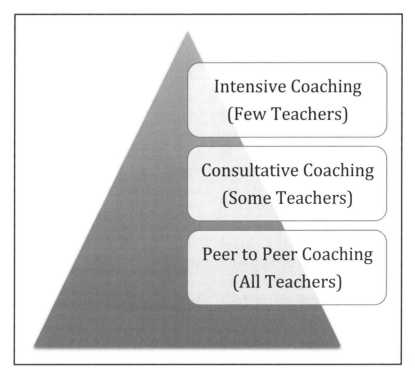

Figure 5–1. Tiered model of coaching support intensity.

Peer-to-peer (PtP) coaching is typically provided on a check-in and as-needed basis. Many teachers with experience implementing evidence-based interventions would be likely to find this level of coaching sufficient in supporting their everyday efforts to effectively teach students with ASDs. Alternatively, some would benefit from a more intensive level of support. Hence, we further elaborate a model called "consultative coaching" at a second tier on the pyramid (see Figure 5–1). Although not intended for all teachers, consultative coaching (CC) would be provided to a select group who may be (a) altogether new to teaching students with ASD;(b) implementing a new program, curriculum, or intervention; or (c) encountering challenges and barriers to successfully implementing specific interventions for a student. Consultative coaching differs in intensity from PtP coaching involving a greater degree of monitoring and support from an outside expert. In-class consultations are provided, and debriefing and follow-up activities are scheduled. Consultative coaching generally consists of a more uniform observation and follow-up schedule than PtP coaching (see expert coaching models described in Chapter 3).

At the top of the coaching pyramid, "intensive" coaching is reserved for a few teachers who would benefit from high-intensity support. In many cases, intensive coaching (IC) will need to be individualized to address the unique needs of the teacher and/or program. There may be many reasons justifying the need for IC. For example, IC would be required when a teacher has insufficient knowledge or background about ASD as a disability, is struggling to be successful in his or her current assignment, and/or, in some cases, is in jeopardy of removal. Intensive coaching may be provided when other problems arise as well, including but not limited to high rates of challenging student behavior, poor collaboration among related service providers, family members, and parent advocates, or other stakeholders who disagree with a teaching methodology, or Individualized Education Program (IEP) goal priorities for a student. Intensive coaching may be implemented proactively to enhance the likelihood of success in at-risk situations. Examples might include, but are not limited to, a teacher's first month on the job, the adoption of a new evidence-based program, and/or the introduction of a high-needs student with ASD into an existing program.

Intensive coaching entails direct levels of support where the coach operates as "expert trainer." This level of coaching is the most labor-intensive process, most embedded in terms of the involvement of the coach, and accordingly, the most costly. The coach may be on site in the classroom for a duration of several consecutive school days, conducting observations of instruction and student management, reviewing curriculum resources and materials, and utilizing direct observational tools to record a teacher's differentiated instructional

techniques in the classroom as well as recording students' responses. In many cases, when informed parent consent is obtained, there may be opportunity to video-record the classroom or a particular student for later review and analysis with the teacher and staff. Educational staff serving students with ASD with significant learning, social-communication, and/or behavioral issues may require this level of assistance from a knowledgeable expert to implement instructional change and/or behavioral support.

In many school agencies, related special education support personnel (e.g., speech-language pathologists [SLPs], occupational therapists [OTs], and inclusion specialists) assume the role of consultative coach for higher-functioning students on the autism spectrum included in general education programs. As more SLPs, OTs, and behavior intervention managers enter the special educational work force, there may be an expectation for them to take on broader roles of co-teaching and expert coaching in programs, as well as training team members and other professionals in best practices for the ASD population. The expansion of roles and responsibilities, and the trend away from segregated service delivery models toward inclusive classroom models by well-trained service providers is an evolving practice that requires role release and discipline sharing (see McGinty & Justice, 2007). For example, in addition to imparting a particular expertise in a given specialty of focus, such as augmentative and alternative communication (AAC), school-based SLPs actively model and teach

AAC strategies to the educational team that engages with a student throughout the school day. In a similar vein, instructional assistants (paraprofessionals) can serve as peer coaches for novice instructional aides in classrooms. Coaching is not a role we perceive as belonging to the elite few in the field of special education. Rather, we envision that it will emerge as a transdisciplinary practice in public school systems invested in "cross-pollinating" best practices and implementing interventions that are effective for students on the autism spectrum.

Determining the most appropriate coaching approach requires an understanding of student and teacher needs, and how best to address those needs while allocating district resources. With a three-tiered coaching model, professionals can better direct and provide targeted assistance where and when it is most needed. Unfortunately, sometimes coaching can be inconsistent, and the coachee feels underappreciated, unsupported, and overwhelmed by the additional requirements that a coach places on him or her. This issue was previously previewed in Chapter 1 as "obstacles to coaching." Once a coach clarifies his or her role by undertaking a level of coaching intensity consistent with the needs of the teacher or classroom situation (context), the coachee then has a clearer picture of what to expect, and can enter into a reciprocal problem-solving relationship with the coach. Clarifying the what, why, and where of coaching by utilizing one of these approaches reduces anxiety and increases trust between both parties, which is a key feature of high-quality coaching.

The Autism Services Coach

The increasing need for effective instruction with students with ASD has spawned a new professional title known in many states as an "autism services coach." These individuals receive advanced training from professional organizations or agencies in evidence-based practices and share this information with educational teams. Around the country, networks of professional autism services coaches and trainers (e.g., the California Autism and Professional Training Information Network [CAPTAIN]) offer extended training and on-site consultation to their local educational agencies). The autism services coach provides assistance at any of the levels of support depicted in Figure 5–1. Much of what this professional shares revolves around new practices in the field to ensure that teachers and staff are up-to-date on the latest pedagogies and evidence-based practices for students. The autism services coach appointed by the school district or intermediate-level educational agency (e.g., county office, regional consortium, or collaborative) holds the requisite skill set to assume this expert role. An autism services coach's skill repertoire encompasses knowledge about the neurology and core deficits unique to ASD as well as evaluation and assessment, explicit instructional approaches, data collection, social communication and social skill training, writing and developing IEPs, just to name a few. The job of this expert is to observe, guide, model, and offer ongoing feedback and support, and, most important, demonstrate best educational practices. Across all levels of coaching support, the autism services coach schedules observation time with the teacher and then embeds an organized regimen of support for teacher and other team members and related support services personnel, such as the SLP, OT, the school psychologist, and behavior management specialist. Additionally, the coach develops an action plan helping teachers strive to master strategies that have direct and immediate impact on student academic achievement and functional performance (see Chapter 4, Table 4–2).

Peer-to-Peer (PtP) Coaching

As Figure 5–1 illustrates, the most basic level of coaching support is peer-to-peer (PtP) coaching. Some classrooms that serve students with ASD have credentialed teachers who may or may not have an extensive training background working with students with this disability. A teacher on reassignment may find him- or herself in the position of working in a classroom or program in which they have some, though not expert, experience. Most of these teachers have to learn on the job, be intuitive, and trust their instincts. They end up coaching themselves by initiating discussions with a respected peer or other staff member seeking guidance and support for their instructional decisions. Peer-to-peer coaching is just that, professionals checking in with each other

frequently to dialogue about students with sometimes intense social, behavior, and/or academic needs. This coaching model relies heavily on reciprocal communication, openness to exchanging feedback, and a willingness to make instructional changes. Ultimately, the more experienced partner assumes the role of peer coach or guide, taking time to focus attention on a specific aspect of the classroom or program that the other teacher requests help with. An effective peer coach takes the time to listen and understand why the teacher's instruction is unsuccessful or needs improvement and involves the teacher in identifying problems and solutions. Aside from the informality of this coaching approach, PtP coaching cannot happen effectively "on the fly." There must be time set aside for professionals to discuss classroom organization and make timely and important decisions about students. With time appropriated for decision making, novice teachers can begin to implement, even at a rudimentary level, some of the more advanced concepts or instructional strategies typically found at an intensive or supportive coaching level described below. For instance, it is customary for data to be collected on certain students with behavioral challenges. Educational team members can then to begin to notice changes in behavior from baseline and to make programmatic adjustments reflecting on changes in that data (see Chapter 8).

Peer-to-peer coaching, in many ways, relies on encouragement to prompt teacher improvement. The upside of this coaching model is that it is non-threatening and "group think" in nature; the act of a peer helping another peer builds camaraderie. A feeling that you are in this together makes a difference for teachers in generating a culture of respect and trust. Table 5–1 depicts "key" activities and elements of PtP coaching.

The vignette in Box 5–1 illustrates PtP coaching for a beginning teacher who has little background working with students with ASD and also shows the limitations of this level of support with respect to its long-term effectiveness.

For this teacher and many like her, PtP coaching is akin to being on a lifeboat waiting for a miracle to happen. It would be far better had the school district provided an autism services coach at an intensive coaching level from the very start. Peer-to-peer coaching as a survival approach only goes so far. This level of support is best used as a collaborative method to improve instruction. It is not a suggested coaching model for novice teachers lacking a foundation in the core characteristics of ASD and, more importantly, who lack any prior instructional experience with this population.

Table 5–1. Peer-to-Peer Coaching Checklist

A "peer" coach does the following:

- Uses *attentive listening* when discussing classroom issues
- Focuses attention on any specific aspect of another peer's concern, interest, or performance in a supportive and positive manner
- Confers with the peer on issues to be discussed and encourages different ideas and different perspectives
- Takes the time to understand the issue at hand, and why performance is successful or needs improvement
- Observes the peer's work and solicits feedback from others, if appropriate
- Involves the peer in identifying successes and solutions
- Discusses alternative solutions
- Recognizes and reinforces successes and improvements
- Discusses and agrees on action(s) to be taken
- Develops an Action Plan
- Schedules follow-up meeting(s) to measure results via e-mail, phone, and face-to-face meetings
- Holds each other accountable to report on progress, or lack thereof
- Reflects collaboratively on what strategies work, and what has not worked

---

Box 5–1. Vignette: "Sink or Swim"

Janice received a voicemail from the principal of Hope School on Friday asking her if she wanted to take over a class of upper elementary students with ASD who were housed in a portable at a local elementary school. Janice, who holds an elementary school credential, has been seeking a third-grade teaching position but to no avail. She has no special education training, save for a mandatory introductory class on special needs children in her credentialing program. In a burst of excitement she called the human resource office and agreed to take the position. Well, you can guess what happened in the first week of instruction: Janice was overwhelmed and woefully unprepared. Her check-in coaching occurred with her instructional assistants (IAs) after recess, after lunch, and after school, where she desperately tried to tap into their knowledge. The IAs had been with the class for over 2 years. They were most patient with Janice and understood that she did not have the requisite skills, or even the basic background to work with students with ASD.

During the first month, Janice practiced peer-to-peer coaching daily with the IAs, with the school psychologist, when she could catch him, the SLP, who provided service in the classroom three times a week, and the adapted physical education teacher, all of whom gave her tips and strategies that she incorporated into her lessons. She attended workshops, enrolled in a special education program at the university, and searched every autism website possible. Will she survive the semester?

Peer-to-Peer Coaching Example

Another vignette (Box 5–2) applies the key components of PtP coaching as outlined in the Peer-to-Peer Checklist (see Table 5–1). This case example is emblematic of how peers can coach and support one another using good communication and problem-solving skills.

Box 5–2. Vignette: A Friend in Need

I am a resource specialist at Capitol High School outside of Washington, DC. I have a student, Peter, with ASD who functions fairly well in two content classes with assistance from Ms. Castilino, his one-to-one instructional assistant. Ms. Castilino shared a concern regarding Peter's anxiety about passing the high school benchmark tests. She also indicated that several of the resource program students had the same concerns and had given up on passing the test. To address those concerns, Ms. Castilino asked the students to take out their old exams, worksheets, essays, and previous study guides to review them for the benchmark exam.

After conferring with Ms. Castilino, I suggested that we set up a study group that Ms. Castilino would conduct with Peter and other resource program students needing assistance. I shared several test-taking strategies with Ms. Castilino. I also incorporated her suggestion of collecting as many past exams and worksheets as possible. We launched the study group and agreed that I would observe the group on the second day so that Ms. Castilino could feel comfortable implementing the approach. After the second day, we would discuss the viability of the approach.

In our debriefing session, Ms. Castilino indicated that she had students order their work assignments from the beginning of the quarter to the end. She also had them make an outline of what information they would study each day. Breaks were encouraged and granted so that students learned the value of reducing their test anxiety. On the second day, she asked students what accommodations their general education teachers provided that helped them pass the benchmark exam. The students said that these teachers were pretty supportive and shared this information.

We work at our own pace, and the teachers say that we need to learn every bit of detail that is covered in class. If lecture notes have not been written, or if the teacher is moving too fast, the teacher will take a screen shot of the notes and post them on an Internet portal for the class. We are able to have access to the portal the last 10 minutes of class, and e-mail any notes we missed to ourselves. We are able to go to the learning center and take as long as we need to take the test. Depending on our IEPs, we can access our notes if needed.

I asked Ms. Castilino to identify successes along with potential solutions to any problems that she might anticipate. She indicated that Peter was hesitant to respond in the group; that he sometimes required 30 seconds or more to formulate his thoughts. I asked her how the other students responded to Peter, and she said they are very patient with him. Once he gets going, he asks some very good questions and contributes to the discussion. I suggested we ask Angela, who gets along with Peter, to review the sample tests and assignments with him. I also suggested that Ms. Castilino give positive social feedback when students applied test-taking strategies. Making this a fun experience will help reduce the anxiety for Peter and probably for the rest of the students as well.

We discussed filling out an action plan; however, Ms. Castilino and I thought that with the ideas that were generated and the support the students were receiving from their general education teachers, that progress was underway. I acknowledged Ms. Castilino for her organization and resourcefulness. We both agreed to a check-in at the end of week to make any needed adjustments, to check progress, and to discuss what did not work so well, and what needed to be modified.

Consultative Coaching (CC)

An intermediate level of coaching that provides more intensive support than PtP assistance is consultative coaching (CC). Rather than intermittent "check-ing-in" by the peer/consultant, the CC approach is characterized by frequent scheduled observations and preplanned follow-up activities between an expert coach and coachee. The consultative coach provides an extra set of eyes and ears to help the teaching staff quickly assess the big picture in a classroom. Following an initial classroom observation, the coach overviews the classroom supports and instructional strategies that are effectively working in the program, suggesting modifications that can immediately affect student change. Coach and coachee debrief, and the coach lends insight about specific students and their learning challenges helping the coachee prioritize next steps for implementing instructional change. For example, the coach may suggest that a daily classroom schedule be explicitly reviewed with students at the beginning of the school day and be made visually accessible in written or graphical form at students' desks. A visual schedule is designed to direct students to the structure of the day, to guide their ability to anticipate what is coming next, and to enable them to transition across tasks/ activities independently.

Consultative coaching may evolve over three stages: immediate, mid-range, and long term. During the immediate stage, the coach and teacher identify a pressing issue and drive for a solution with immediate benefit to the student and the teacher. Mid-range and long-term solutions involve crafting changes to the classroom instruction that take more time to implement, typically where extended follow-up visits are required by the coach. The CC process we describe comes closest to functional models of consultation known as a "collaborative" that have strong support among educational researchers. Others have emphasized the importance of requisite interpersonal communica-

tion and problem-solving skills of the consultative coach (Idol, Paoloucci-Whitcomb, & Nevin, 2000; Kampwirth, 2006; Kucharczyk, Shaw, Smith-Myles, Sullivan, Szidon, & Tuchman-Ginsberg, 2012; Rush, Shelden, & Raab, 2008); these interpersonal and professional traits were addressed in Chapters 1 and 2. Key elements of the consultative process are summarized in Table 5–2.

There are a variety of structured ways for coaches to record ongoing notes about classroom instruction and student behavior. In Table 5–3, the coach begins by listing the names of the students and adults, as well as sketching an overall floor plan of the physical arrangement of the classroom with notation about where students sit relative to each other, where primary instruction occurs, and how and where instruction is delivered in the classroom. Language arts instruction, for example, may occur in small learning groups at a side table; alternatively, math instruction might be delivered to the entire class at the front of the room.

At the top of the page in Table 5–3, a record is made of the classroom schedule as it appears on the teacher's lesson plan or displayed within the room. As observation begins, it is helpful to record both the start and stop times of the lesson or activity. This information will be important for later teacher feedback about the duration of instruction and ongoing student behavior. It is also helpful for the coach as a memory tool when observation happens for a partial day of instruction. Finally, a brief narrative of teacher instructions, what

Table 5–2. Consultative Coaching Checklist

The consultative coach does the following:

- Schedules a plan for classroom observation and discusses issues teacher would like input on

- Practices active listening; lets the teacher speak first about her or his needs, what she or he would most like support with, and what she or he perceives as challenges/problems

- Arrives at the start of a designated activity time; stays initially focused on the big picture

- Collects objective assessment: written notes, checklists/forms, recordings (video) for later analysis

- Schedules a follow-up time; this may be during lunch or recess time for the coachee(s)

- Solicits opinions about whether student behavior or performance in the observed activity was typical or "atypical," and if the latter, asks about factors that might explain unrepresentative behavior from student(s)

- Encourages coachee(s) to discover what must be changed and why

- Uses a combination of objective assessment sharing (notes, recordings, rating scales, etc.) and individualized coaching sessions to help coachee(s) address skill gaps, define personal goals, develop an action plan, and monitor progress toward those goals

- Suggests practical interventions and strategies; may volunteer to create or reproduce needed materials or resources

- Returns to classroom for follow-up observation and team visitations

- Recognizes a consultee's successes and improvements

- Schedules follow-up meeting(s) to discuss outcomes

- Works collaboratively to eliminate barriers to reaching objectives

students are doing and/or saying, and so on, is transcribed by the coach during the observation. As student learning or classroom challenges occur, written notation may follow; for example, a prescription symbol (Rx) in Table 5–3 identifies an explicit intervention or strategy that the coach feels would correct or augment a skill or expected behavior from the student, such as, defining a social rule in a social script or narrative.

Consultative Coaching (CC) Case Example

Roberto is an elementary school student with high-functioning autism capable

Table 5–3. Sample Consultative Coaching Observation Notes

Inclusion Class—Second Grade—Abraham School	
Teacher	Mary Ellen Montague (MM)
Instructional Assistants	Lee C. (LC) and Travis M.
Students	25 General Education second-grade students + 2 students with IEPs: Roberto M., and Taylor W.
[Classroom floor plan goes here; sketch of essential landmarks and locations]	
Daily Schedule	
Morning Meeting	8:20–8:35
English Language Arts (ELA): Daily Journal	8:35–9:00
Reading Groups	9:00–9:45
Math (Calculation)	9:45–10:10
Recess	10:10–10:30
Math (Application)	10:30–11:00
ELA: Reading/Writing	11:00–11:40
Lunch	11:40–12:35
Science/Computer Lab (M-W-F)	12:35–1:30
Social Skills Training (T-Th)	12:35–1:30
Social Studies (M-W-F)	1:30–2:00
P.E. (T-Th)	1:30–2:00
Recess	2:00–2:15
Homework Assignments	2:15–2:35
Dismissal	2:40
Observation	9:45–10:10 AM: Daily Math Calculation worksheets (Lesson 5—Subtraction: Regrouping 2-digit numbers). Three students (Ian, Emily, Roberto) are working independently at their desks with base-10 blocks. Roberto: Writes name, begins worksheet, stops at item #8, puts head down on desktop, does not reorient to task, and whines when prompted to complete up to item #15 by LC.
Rx	Break down this math assignment into two 10-item worksheets. Visual or auditory timer can be set at 5-minute intervals at Roberto's desk. Show Roberto a visual "pacing" guide. (Guide depicts 5 blank "boxes" to be checked every 3 minutes of task completion.) Guide has graphics for "keep working," "when finished," and "choose an activity." For every 3 minutes of successful "on-task" worksheet calculation, Roberto gives himself a check mark (✓). When 5 ✓ are achieved, Roberto gets to choose a "preferred break" activity.

of completing most daily academic routines, but who often fails to complete in-class work. When assignments are explained, Roberto ultimately gets anxious and will "shut down," giving up after the first few minutes of attempting the assignment. This behavior pattern is extremely frustrating for the inclusion assistant, who finds himself in the role of cajoling Roberto to finish his work. The teacher, Ms. Montague, is a skilled general elementary program teacher with a track record of including students like Roberto in her program. Ms. Montague has attended professional training workshops on supporting students with ASDs and has a history of being flexible with the special education program at her school site, readily accepting students in her class that other teachers decline. Among her successful strategies is a point system and tangible rewards system offered at the end of the week to incentivize students for completed work, but Roberto never seems to get "off the dime." Roberto's behavior is concerning for his educational team as his progress on his academic and behavior IEP goals has stalled. Ms. Montague and the special education coordinator seek specialized coaching assistance from an autism services coach, a program specialist with past experience teaching students with ASD.

The coach calls the teacher and special education (SPED) coordinator to get their description of the challenges facing Roberto and to set up a time for a planned visit to the classroom. The coach further learns that Roberto has transitioned successfully from a self-contained classroom, where he was regarded as the "star" student academically and behaviorally. He is very capable, and his recent psycho-educational assessment indicates that intellectually he performs above average in verbal reasoning and spatial and analytical reasoning. Further, his achievement of academic abilities was well within the range expected for his intelligence. According to the teacher, "when Roberto started in my class, expectations were very high that he would succeed with a minimum of inclusion support because he had few if any behavioral challenges." The coach learned that Roberto's difficulties occur primarily during lessons in which students have to work independently on written tasks. The coach arranged a time and day for her observation of Ms. Montague's class and returned later that week to meet with the teacher and her staff at a time when instruction was over. She asked whether Roberto's behavior of shutting down was "typical" as she began surveying their responses to several open-ended questions about what they thought might be contributing to Roberto's reluctance to finishing the math worksheet. The educational team agreed with the coach's assessment of Roberto: that he has difficulty organizing himself and keeping track of what he has accomplished and what he has left to do. The coach suggested that Roberto appeared overwhelmed by the number of math problems on the page, concluding that he could not power through 20 minutes of independent math calculation problems at his desk.

In this scenario, the coach further shared her Rx, which was to break the assignment into two shorter assignments and to assist Roberto with self-monitoring his own behavior by providing a visual timer, and a visual support guide that he could check off every 3 to 5 minutes while monitoring his on-task behavior. When the requisite number of boxes on the pacing guide was checked, Roberto could then choose a break activity of short duration. Self-monitoring is an evidence-based intervention strategy for students with ASD that has been successfully implemented with school psychologists employing consultative coaching models (Wilkinson, 2005).

Intensive Coaching (IC)

Intensive coaching (IC) occurs at the most involved level of teacher support; this level of coaching consists of high-frequency, high-quality contact between an expert and teacher and is reserved for situations where the deployment of comprehensive resources can more easily be justified. Intensive coaching may best be utilized when sweeping changes in instructional programs are adopted, or when a particular teacher is struggling to deliver effective programming to students. This model could include a coaching regimen wherein the coach provides direct guidance, modeling, and instruction 4 days in 1 week, with day 5 left open for reinforcing the implementation of instructional methods, modi-

fying action plans, and making note of how and when a teacher masters key skills that were modeled or discussed during the week. The coach then tapers support over a period of time (gradual release), so that the teacher can assume responsibility for instruction with check-in times from the coach for reassurance and input.

The coach establishes a schedule with the teacher and other staff so that coaching integrates naturally into the classroom setting. An intensive support coach has to be willing to work with students in the classroom, signaling willingness for shared roles with the teacher for supporting learning, one of the basic tenets of high-quality coaching. The coach also models strategies that she or he wants the teacher or staff to incorporate into instruction. Reciprocal communication as outlined in Chapter 4 is the basis for this type of intensive coaching. The following weekly coaching schedule highlights the intensity of this approach.

Day 1: Autism services coach reviews IEP documents and, on an electronic tablet or laptop computer, reviews key IEP goals for students that coach and teacher will target. If there are general classroom goals, such as engineering the physical arrangement of the room, then the coach will identify those areas of need. The coach spends an entire day in observation getting to know the culture and dynamic of the classroom, determining how students interact with the teacher and staff.

Day 2: The autism services coach spends the full day working directly or indirectly with students in the classroom identifying learning and behavior challenges. The coach keys in on two or three students who may need explicit instruction to support their stated IEP goals. For example, coach and teacher determine which students may require a prompt fading procedure to master the selected skills. The teacher may be unsure about where and when to teach a skill and how to monitor student progress in response to the fading of prompts. In the debriefing session at the end of the day, the coach and teacher decide on how best to focus instruction to help the identified students. The coach shares a Task Analytic Data Form (see Chapter 8, Table 8–6) and an Instructional Setting Evaluation Form (see Chapter 9, Table 9–1), aimed at monitoring instruction. If appropriate, the coach can offer suggestions regarding additional progress monitoring forms, such as those in Chapter 8.

Day 3: The coach and teacher implement some of their discussed ideas related to explicit instruction with the class as a whole, noting the impact of an instructional strategy for students needing more support. The coach notes the type of prompting the teacher uses to get a sense of what might be the best approach to use for any particular student requiring this support.

Day 4: After debriefing (see Day 2), the coach and teacher initially reverse roles with the coach modeling explicit instruction with the whole class, while the teacher monitors student behavior and task performance. The coach then has the teacher practice explicit instruction, observes once again, and provides feedback. This sequence is repeated one more time if time allows.

Day 5: The coach and the teacher collaboratively develop an action plan using the Action Plan Worksheet (Table 5–4) for the next week. For example, fading a prompt procedure with a particular student might be part of the plan. Both parties work together filling out the Action Plan determining what each member and other classroom staff will do to accomplish the plan.

This 5-day intensive coaching model with an expert coach and a receptive teacher promotes classroom success. The times and days for intense coaching can be modified based on need. Whatever way that IC is delivered, it must be well organized, and coaches must be considerate of teacher and curriculum time demands in order for this concentrated approach to be embraced. The impact of this type of coaching can be significant resulting in long-lasting change in teacher skills, classroom management, and individual student behavior. This approach requires a coach to follow up regularly and often with coachee(s)

Table 5–4. Action Plan Worksheet for Coaches and Teachers

Action Plan Worksheet: From Vision to Action		
Today's Date:		
Purpose of Action Plan:		
WHO	**Will do WHAT**	**By WHEN/Status**

to ensure mastery and maintenance of skills (Tables 5–5 and 5–6).

Teachers may have myriad resources at their disposal, yet be unable to take advantage of this type of support because they are overwhelmed, anxious, or unprepared. Coaches need to be aware of the demeanor of the teacher and the classroom environment they are entering. One must be cognizant of the minute-to-minute changes that happen in a classroom; one behavioral incident from a student can disrupt the flow of instruction. With all levels of coaching support discussed here, coaches and related personnel assigned to a classroom must be extra responsive to some of the stressors that confront teachers and classroom staff on a day-to-day basis. It behooves every coach to be patient, creating the context for change through supportive communication and relationship building, providing opportunities for actionable change in the classroom.

Table 5–5. Intensive Coaching Checklist

Learn
• Observe the class for the first day, jotting down notes.
• Observe and interact with other professionals and students on Day 2 and take mental and written notes.
• Debrief with the teacher and other professionals at key times during the first two days.
• Be mindful of and use effective interpersonal communication when interacting with the consultee (see Communication Demeanor, Chapter 4).
• Share your experiences to help the consultee feel accepted.
• Understand your strengths and weaknesses as a coach, and be clear about your own boundaries as well as the boundaries of your role as a coach.
• Maintain a positive mental attitude toward oneself as coach and toward the person you are coaching (see Positive Attitude, Chapter 4).
• Have strategic and focused conversations using reciprocal communication techniques, especially Attentive Listening (Chapter 4).
• Stay in touch with the reality your consultee is facing.
• Identify a few goals to work on for the remainder of the first week.
• Create a time schedule with the consultee for more intensive coaching with feedback and debriefing sessions.
• Move into the analyze stage of intensive coaching.

Analyze
• Use multiple data collection and analysis techniques to guide intervention strategies or methods. Identify forms to use and refer to these throughout the coaching sessions (see Chapter 8).
• Solicit feedback from the consultee during coaching sessions.
• Utilize daily coaching logs and debrief at predetermined checkpoints during the day (for example, 60% classroom based and 40% teacher conferences at end of the day).
• Strive for mastery via demonstration lessons, co-teaching, and/or direct feedback.
• Conduct weekly coaching meetings with consultee and other team members.
• Connect the data gathered to an Action Plan (see Table 5–4 above).
• Document increased levels of teaching competency.
• Provide specific and measurable results that the consultee can identify and attest to the effectiveness of (see Strategy Check in Table 5–6).

Grow
• To build trust, avoid inactivity in the classroom; stay engaged with an ongoing lesson, the students, or the teaching staff.
• Frequently follow through with consultee(s).
• Do not promise more than you can deliver.
• Do not hide your ignorance; ask questions.
• Celebrate successes along the way.

Table 5–6. Coaching Strategy Check

I assessed the need for selecting the strategy.	YES	NO
I explained the rationale for using the strategy.	YES	NO
I defined the strategy.	YES	NO
I explained to another adult when to use the strategy.	YES	NO
I modeled the strategy.	YES	NO
I provided other examples for the student.	YES	NO
I debriefed with another adult about the strategy.	YES	NO
I reminded a student to use the strategy.	YES	NO

Summary

A coaching framework is developed in this chapter with three levels of high-quality coaching that are differentiated on the basis of their intensity of support. All are designed to help improve instructional effectiveness in programs for students with ASD. The least intensive level of support, peer-to-peer coaching, is invoked when the goal is to support instruction without allocating the resources of an outside expert or "autism services" coach. When more intensive support is required, consultative and/or intensive coaching levels are indicated. Context and need dictate which of these types of coaching is more appropriate for a teacher and/or educational staff. All three support levels are collaborative and require key attributes of high-quality coaching introduced in previous chapters of this book. Embedding coaching in the classroom where professionals can make decisions in the natural teaching environment makes a discernable difference in instructional effectiveness, student progress, and teacher self-efficacy.

End-of-Chapter Questions

1. There are three levels of coaching identified in this chapter. In your own words, describe each of the coaching models. Which one of the coaching models do you use or are you most familiar with, and why? Which of the coaching models would be of greatest help to you right now and why? Can you see the value of all three models? Explain your answer in detail. Make sure to indicate whether your school district or local educational agency provides coaching in the way it is outlined here or a variation of what this chapter describes.

2. Write a letter to your school administrator about the importance of

providing consultative and intensive coaching to better serve students with ASD. Do not request contracting with an outside agency for coaching support. Your assignment here is to request internal district support from an autism services coach, or other district interventionist (e.g., program specialist) with the requisite skills to coach you. Make sure you use the information found in this chapter to develop a cogent rationale (specify your reasons) for your request, and that you nail down a coaching schedule for either consultative or intensive coaching.

3. You have just been asked by your school district to apply for a "high-quality coach-autism" position. After reading this chapter, and more specifically, the section on the autism services coach, write a good justification for why you might be well suited for the job. (This is an exercise to encourage you to think about the characteristics of an expert coach serving students with ASD.) You must include a justification of your reasons based on what you have read thus far in Section I. Plan on writing approximately a page or page and a half. Make sure the letter has a formal convincing tone without boasting, or over selling yourself. NOTE: For many of you currently working with an autism services coach, use this as an opportunity to discuss areas of improvement.

4. Identify a situation in your classroom or in a hypothetical classroom

where a teacher could benefit from one of the coaching models: peer-to-peer, consultative, or intensive coaching. Assume the role of the coach and follow the steps on the checklist for the model you choose. Make sure that you make a clear plan with measurable outcomes for the teacher you are coaching. This activity is meant to be enjoyable because you are actually coaching yourself and, possibly, a few members of your instructional team. Be creative, honest, and use this activity to identify an issue that you have wanted to tackle.

5. Review Table 5–5 and identify a strategy you would like to use in your classroom or are presently implementing. Apply the steps in the Strategy Check from Table 5–6. Oftentimes, coaches tell teachers about strategies or send them to a website but do not demonstrate or model the strategy. As a coach it is imperative that, if indeed you suggest a strategy, you model it and/or provide resources to make it possible for implementation.

References

Cramer, S. F. (1998). *Collaboration: A success strategy for special educators*. Boston, MA: Allyn & Bacon.

Idol, L., Paoloucci-Whitcomb, P., & Nevin, A. (2000). *Collaborative consultation*. Austin, TX: Pro-Ed.

Kampwirth, T. J. (2006). *Collaborative consultation in the schools: Effective practices for students with learning and behavior problems* (3rd ed.). Upper Saddle River, NJ: Pearson.

Kampwirth, T. J., & Powers, K. M. (2011). *Collaborative consultation in the schools: Effective practices for students with learning and behavior problems* (4th ed.). Upper Saddle River, NJ: Pearson.

Kucharczyk, S., Shaw, E., Smith Myles, B., Sullivan, L., Szidon, K., & Tuchman-Ginsberg, L. (2012). *Guidance and coaching on evidence-based practices for learners with autism spectrum disorders.* Chapel Hill, NC: University of North Carolina, Frank Porter Graham Child Development Institute, National Professional Development Center on Autism Spectrum Disorders.

McGinty, A. S., & Justice, L. (2007). Classroom-based versus pull-out intervention: A review of the experimental evidence. *Autism Internet Modules EBP Briefs, 1,* 1–14.

Rush, D. D., Shelden, M. L., & Raab, M. (2008). A framework for reflective questioning when using a coaching interaction style. *CASEtools: Instruments and Procedures for Implementing Early Childhood and Family Support Practices, 4*(1), 1–7.

Wilkinson, L. A. (2005). Supporting the inclusion of a student with Asperger syndrome: A case study using conjoint behavioral consultation and self-management. *Educational Psychology in Practice, 21*(4), 307–326.

SECTION II

Using High-Quality Coaching in Planning Instruction for Students With Autism Spectrum Disorder

Section II complements Section I by illustrating how the High-Quality Coaching–Autism (HQC-A) model can be utilized in supporting teachers to plan for the instruction of students with ASD. The section details the roles and responsibilities of a collaborative team in regard to the special education process and how coaches can be active participants. The section also provides specifics about how coaches can assist educators in understanding how assessment informs instruction, and how to establish progress monitoring practices at the outset of program delivery to ensure the effectiveness of instruction.

CHAPTER 6

Using High-Quality Coaching to Support Collaborative Teaming

Never doubt that a small group of thoughtful, committed citizens
can change the world; indeed, it's the only thing that ever has.

—Margaret Mead

Chapter Objectives

- Assist coaches and teachers in working with a team to support the skill development of students with autism spectrum disorder (ASD).

- Provide tips for recruiting family involvement and collaborating with family members.

- Provide information on key roles and members of collaborative teams.

- Present key considerations on how to run team meetings.

- Provide ideas for enhancing collaborative efforts among team members.

Introduction

You have certainly heard the saying, "It takes a village." When it comes to educating students with autism spectrum disorder, this saying could not be more relevant. The coaching relationship we have discussed thus far is an excellent start toward building a collaborative team focused on identifying meaningful goals and providing effective instruction and supports for these students. However, actually identifying, recruiting, and effectively collaborating with others for the purpose of teaching social communicative skills, or addressing behavior concerns may be an area in which new and veteran teachers will need support from a high-quality coach. Coaches can support teachers by providing and seeking out answers to the following questions: "Who should be on the team?" "When, where, and how often should we meet?" "How can I effectively facilitate team meetings?" "How do we keep our focus on the needs of the child?" This chapter provides guidance on many of these questions, and further information will likely need to be obtained and addressed given the unique features of each district, school, and team. The coach can serve an instrumental role in working with the teacher to provide this information and to seek out additional details and resources to support the functioning of an effective team. The vignette described in Box 6–1 illustrates a far too common scenario in which educational professionals and family members find themselves when the collaborative process is not in place.

Rationale

In the regular hustle and bustle of typical school settings and while working with individuals with a variety of personalities and potential interpersonal issues, pausing to brainstorm, collaborate, and check in with one another seems like a luxury coaches cannot achieve or afford. However, research tells us that when instructional programs are developed through careful planning and collaboration with key stakeholders, it results in better outcomes for students with ASD (National Research Council, 2001). Because deficits in social interaction impact so many in the child's environment, multiple partners may need to participate in this process. Given the multifaceted social-communicative and behavior needs that children with ASD face, it is crucial that individuals with varied expertise and perspectives be involved in the identification and selection of meaningful goals and strategies to effectively address these needs. Furthermore, when people who know the student well are involved in the identification of goals and the selection of strategies, these programs possess what professionals in the field refer to as "contextual relevance" (McLaughlin, Denney, Snyder, & Welsh, 2012). Contextual relevance or "contextual fit" refers to the match between the strategies selected, and the skill sets and comfort level of those who will be implementing them (Crone & Horner, 2003). Thus, when individuals are involved in the identification and selection of instructional and other support strategies, those

---

Box 6–1. Vignette: Communication Breakdown

Jennifer walked into the meeting with her coach, Brian, and began to share her concerns about collaborating with the family of one of her students. Jennifer's student, Brianna, spends her day in a general education third-grade class with her peers, and Jennifer provides additional supports to her in that setting. Even though Brianna's mother and the general education teacher had never really "clicked," over the past few months their relationship has rapidly deteriorated. Brianna's mother and the general education teacher had recently engaged in multiple verbal sparring matches during morning drop-off and afternoon pickup times. During these altercations, a few "choice words" were said in front of both students and other staff. The general education teacher reported these incidents to the principal, who successfully obtained a restraining order against Brianna's mother prohibiting her from setting foot on school grounds. Just that morning, Jennifer had received an e-mail from Brianna's father, an attorney, who was legally separated from Brianna's mother and shared custody of Brianna. He wanted to know when Brianna's annual IEP meeting would be held. In his e-mail he informed Jennifer that if a meeting was not held prior to the expiration date of her current annual IEP next month, he would be pursuing due process against the district. Jennifer told Brian, "I love working with Brianna, and she's making great progress, but how in the world am I supposed to work with these adults?"

---

participants as actual stakeholders are more likely to be comfortable in using them, leading to a greater impact for the student.

When it comes to supporting and promoting the development of skills for students with ASD, the primary context for teaming would be the Individualized Education Program (IEP) team. The purpose of the IEP team is to develop and oversee the implementation of the student's IEP, which would include educational services and goals related to that particular student's skills.

Who Should Be Involved?

Coaches can assist the teacher at all three levels of coaching (peer-to-peer, consultative coaching, and intensive coaching) in determining who to recruit and involve when assembling a team to support the development and implementation of evidence-based programs for children with ASD. When assembling a team, the key consideration is to select individuals who know the student(s) and the school, and classroom conditions well. Thus, general and special education teachers, instructional assistants, related service providers such as speech-language clinicians, occupational therapists, behavior consultants, and district administrators should all be considered. Additionally, when focusing on programming for an individual student, every effort should be made to include and support the participation of the student's parents. The Individuals with Disabilities Education Improvement Act (IDEIA, 2004) provides guidelines regarding who must be included on the IEP team; however, it is important that the teacher, ideally with the support of at least a consultative coach, actively recruits and welcomes each team member to ensure that this collaborative planning process fulfills not only the letter of the law but also the true spirit of the law. With regard to the coach and teacher relationship, an ideal arrangement would be for the coach to be directly supported by the district, in turn supporting the teacher with consultative, or if necessary, intensive coaching to facilitate the IEP team. The coach may need to provide resources, advice, and even modeling of how to facilitate team meetings. This would provide for enhanced consistency between the broader district-level planning and the on-site implementation of effective programming for students with ASD.

Collaborating With Families

It is crucial to continuously keep in mind the fact that family members are the most important individuals in the lives of children with ASD. They are the true experts when it comes to their child (Dunlap, Newton, Fox, Benito, & Vaughn, 2001). Besides the child, parents are the ones who will be most affected by the strategies implemented as part of the student's educational program. Coaches can support teachers in reaching out to parents in a positive and constructive manner, and in restoring partnerships with parents when contentious relationships have developed. Textbooks have been written entirely on this topic alone (e.g., Smith, Gartin, Murdick, & Hilton, 2006; Turnbull, Turnbull, Erwin, Soodak, & Shogren, 2011), but some of the common themes identified in this important area are briefly summarized in Table 6–1.

Parents often seek information about their child's daily behavior and performance from educational staff and, thus, request ongoing communication from educational staff. Sending notes home to parents is a key communication component, which on a daily basis necessitates that the teacher or other support staff member understands how and what to say, how to write in a clear and consistent manner, and to remain open to parental feedback. Communicating with parents about what transpires during the day makes a difference in the home life of students. Parents, the child's first teachers, often use the information to assist their child at home and

Table 6–1. Coaching Tips for Collaborating With Families

Coaching tips for establishing a family-friendly team environment	Greet parents in a friendly, courteous manner.
	Use name tags for initial meetings.
	Introduce team members to family members and have them briefly describe their role in relationship to supporting the student.
	Ask parents to provide photos of student with friends and family to share during meetings.
	Invite parents to observe class at an appropriate activity and time of the school day.
Coaching tips for communicating effectively	Send messages home consistently and frequently.
	Use a high ratio of specific positive comments to negative comments/concerns.
	Use "I statements" when discussing sensitive or emotional topics.

	Use active listening techniques	Orient posture toward parents when they are speaking.
		Rephrase their statements and ask a follow-up question to show you understand them.
		Avoid trying to talk parents out of their feelings.
		Allow parents to speak without interruption.
		Refrain from offering solutions when parents express being upset; instead, acknowledge feelings and provide supportive statements.

Coaching tips for enhancing cultural sensitivity and competence	Learn about other cultures' values, attitudes, manners, and views.
	Know and respect the religious holidays and observances of the student's family.
	Invite parents to talk about their cultural or ethnic practices.
	Provide written communication in the family's preferred language.
	Ask if parents would like to have a translator present during meetings.
Coaching tips for defusing difficult situations	Listen carefully and respectfully. Refrain from responding until the parent has said everything she or he has to say. Often, just having been listened to by an education professional can result in a family member feeling that the problem has been solved.
	Apologize if you were wrong, or simply for the fact that there is a problem.
	Focus discussion on common areas of agreement and what can be done (rather than on what cannot be accomplished).
	Identify and clarify issues among parents and team members that are pending or need closure.

continues

Table 6–1. *continued*

Coaching tips for defusing difficult situations *continued*	Have the team notetaker log on chart paper what these mutual agreements are, and visually display this during the meeting.
	Alternatively, use another piece of paper to put in a "parking lot" issues that need to be deferred or delayed for later action.
	If agreement is not possible, schedule a follow-up meeting and/or invite others to provide input on resolving the problem.
Coaching tips for strengthening family partnerships	Avoid entering a helper-helpee relationship with parents, and instead seek to establish relationships with parents as educational partners (Turnbull, Turnbull, Erwin, Soodak, & Shogren, 2011).
	View family involvement as a goal, rather than a static characteristic of families. Activities to enhance family involvement should be pursued with all families regardless of how much or how little they are actively involved (Smith, Gartin, Murdick, & Hilton, 2006).
	Run effective meetings: begin meetings with time for positive comments, and check in with parents prior to ending the meeting to make sure their issues/concerns have all been addressed.

to address any concerns the parent or teaching team may have. A coach who takes the time to discuss the importance of communicating with parents on a daily basis can model ways to communicate and then follow up with the teacher to ascertain that the skill is implemented and cement the application of this most important communication process (Box 6–2).

A note system or "log" devised by the teacher, with mentoring help if needed, becomes a salient communication tool between school and home. The "Daily Note Home" shown in Table 6–2 gives parents more information about what occurs during the entire school day rather than just concentrating on specific incidents or student behavior. Teachers working with students with ASD need to remember that student behavior, though important, does not always convey the whole picture of what happens in a day at school. Parents who receive pertinent and timely information value the teaching and learning that takes place in the classroom for their children (Kluth, 2009). A related strategy, the "Communication Log Book" (Kluth, 2010) works similarly. With this strategy, both the teacher and parent(s) exchange brief notes about the student's day, and any ongoing concerns at home can be addressed that day in school, or vice versa. For example, if a student had a challenging morning at home before leaving for school, the teacher can be alerted to this fact by the log and make accommodations as needed, so that school staff are sensitive to not putting undue demands on the student first thing in the morning.

In learning how to implement the daily note home, the coach shares the

---

Box 6–2. Vignette: Mr. Zebo Learns a New Skill

Mr. Zebo, an upper elementary special education teacher working with students with ASD, has good rapport with their parents in face-to-face interactions. The parents respect his easygoing style and his positive interactions with their children. The parents have requested some sort of daily communiqué or note in order to reinforce social and academic skills they noticed taking place in the classroom. To that end, Mr. Zebo has been handing out a scribbled note with general comments (e.g., "Sheila had a good day!" with a smiley face) for the students to bring home at the end of the day. Although parents appreciate his attempt to communicate daily, they still feel the need to have a more systematized communication process in place. They definitely want to be an active part of their child's educational team and to do everything possible to help their children develop appropriate social skills prior to entering junior high. Mr. Zebo has access to an autism services coach from the district, who checks in each week and has offered to help him to communicate more effectively with these parents. The coach has talked to him about using the Daily Note Home, a method of daily communication that she has found to be valued by many families with students with ASD.

---

importance of starting off with student accomplishments. Parents are more open to suggestions after reading positive statements about their children. Practicing how to write positive comments and detailing accomplishments is an exercise that should not be left to chance. New activities indicate student willingness and engagement, which are key to parents feeling comfortable with new experiences their children are offered at school. The reader will also note that behavior comes second to last on the Daily Note Home form (see Table 6–2). Verbal and nonverbal communication

attempts from the student might emanate from a daily tally that the instructional assistant keeps and can then be transcribed for the parent. Recorded emotions and feeling words expressed by the student help the parent understand the range of emotional feelings their child exhibits at school, which could be quite different than how he or she expresses him- or herself at home.

Too often, written communication sent home mentions behavioral transgressions leading to parental discouragement. When addressing behavior concerns, it is important that these be

Table 6–2. Daily Note Home

DAILY NOTE HOME for ALAN	Date: 3/23/2015
Accomplishments/ positives	Great day! Alan scored a 5 (Advanced) on the math benchmark assessment. This is a great success. What's better is that I didn't modify or accommodate it in any way. He was jazzed in his wonderful Alan way.
New activities	We introduced Alan to "Co-Writer," a computer program that corrects grammar and spelling mistakes and offers suggestions for rewording written phrases. Like all new activities with Alan, it takes him a bit of time to warm up to them, but I sensed that he liked this. Please come by so we can show it to you.
New verbal and nonverbal communication	He said, "*according*" today. It came out of the blue. His sister must be using some big words at home. Hope he keeps it up.
Behavior	Still working through picking at skin on his forearm. Still charting and will have more information by the end of the week. We don't want to make this into an issue because he is not obsessed with it.
Emotions expressed	Joy over his math grade. Of course we praised him a lot. We are so proud of him!
Concerns	Alan mentioned Disneyland. Wondering if the family is planning a trip or if he is just into Disneyland?

phrased positively and in a solution-oriented fashion in the daily note home. A coach and the teacher should review the notes every 2 weeks for a period of 2 months, so that this skill/activity becomes second nature for the teacher and is sustained. Mastering the skill of sending notes home that are written in a positive and constructive tone requires practice and some degree of oversight from a mentor or coach. In the example above, you will note the way the teacher highlighted the student's accomplishments and other areas on the daily note home.

Working as a Team

Once the team has been assembled, the real work of collaboration begins. Although the benefits to collaboration are clear, it is important to note that many teams fail to reach their potential in effectively serving students when this process breaks down. By planning proactively to prevent any degradation of the team process, coaches and teachers can work together to create an environment where collaborative activities among team members will be conducted effectively. This planning process should involve the following major activities of collaborative teaming: (a) identifying roles and responsibilities, (b) developing and committing to norms of behavior, (c) running effective meetings, and (d) providing opportunities for team members to step outside of their traditional areas of activity (e.g., role release).

Team Member Roles and Responsibilities

In order to function effectively, team members will need to know what is expected in their respective roles. Over time, effective teams have learned that in order to function at their best, a few specific roles and responsibilities will need to be taken on by individual team members.

Team Facilitator

The facilitator is the glue that holds the team together. This role involves coordinating collaborative activities, including team meetings and communication among team members. During meetings, the facilitator leads the team through the agenda by focusing conversation on the topic at hand, reframing off-topic comments to bring the conversation back on topic, and using strategies, such as "parking lots," to keep the team focused on the topics they have agreed to discuss. The "parking lot" strategy involves writing down new ideas generated by team members, which are not related to original meeting agenda items, and postponing them for later discussion

after consensus agenda items have been discussed. Coaches can model ways of positively and effectively interacting with team members during meetings to keep conversation focused on the task at hand.

Timekeeper

Time may very well be the most precious resource in the work of education professionals. As such, scheduling time to meet together as a team may be difficult, resulting in a tight time frame when all members are available. Therefore, it is essential that during team meetings, one team member serves in the role as timekeeper. Specific time frames should be allocated for each agenda item, and the timekeeper will need to give prompts to the team when they are approaching the end of time intervals designated for each item. Letting the team know, for example, that only a minute remains for the given agenda item, and asking whether resolution can be reached, or if the item should be tabled, can help the team navigate through a long agenda. Coaches can work with teachers to allocate reasonable time frames for agenda items, suggest time-keeping strategies (e.g., using an audio or visual timer), and suggest which team member might be recruited to serve as an effective timekeeper.

Notetaker

Have you ever been to a meeting and then afterward wondered why you went? Or what you were supposed to do before the next meeting? Or what was discussed? With so much on everyone's plate these days, keeping a written record of each meeting becomes increasingly important, simply as a survival mechanism. This is particularly important when agreements have been reached, action plans have been developed, and upcoming meetings have been scheduled. For this reason, at each team meeting a team member will need to be tasked with taking notes; notes are an effective way of logging primary agreements as well as tracking issues for which closure is needed (see Table 6–3). With recent advances in technology, this task is becoming increasingly simplified. Notetakers can use electronic versions of the meeting agenda to record minutes using a laptop computer or tablet. Notes can then be e-mailed to team members, or uploaded to a server, or to secure shared files, where all team members have access. The days of running off copies to be placed in staff and faculty boxes in the mailroom are on their way out, if not long gone already.

Snackmaster

This is our favorite team member. In all seriousness, the mere presence of refreshments during a team meeting can have a positive impact on the tone and nature of interactions among team members. Even leaders of warring civilizations will sit down together over food as a signal of when a peace agreement has been reached. What more can we hope for with contentious special education teams? Simple refreshments, like fruit, vegetables, sweets, water, coffee, and so on, can be made available even with the smallest of funds available for this purpose.

Additional Considerations

An important consideration when it comes to team roles and responsibilities is to rotate them. Giving another team member, such as a parent, an opportunity to facilitate a meeting can promote an environment of collegiality. Rotating the timekeeper role among team members avoids any one member getting pegged with the reputation of always cutting off conversation. Rotating the notetaker role reduces the likelihood of one team member developing carpel tunnel syndrome, while rotating the snackmaster role reduces the potential for resentment of other team members freeloading.

Establishing Team Ground Rules for Behavior and Decision Making

The coach and teacher may find that establishing team norms and ground rules for interactions may be beneficial in order to promote and maintain positive, efficient, and effective interactions among all team members. This is particularly important if any previous interactions among any of the team members have been negative or contentious. Ground rules and "team norms" should be reviewed and endorsed by all team members during the first team meeting. These can then be displayed during all future meetings for quick review at the start of each meeting, and referenced when problems occur during the collaborative process. A sampling of possible ground rules might include, "we will treat each other with respect," "all contributions to our discussions will be valued and heard," "one person will speak at a time," "we will start and end meetings on time," "we will use 'I' statements," and so on.

Running a Meeting

Finding sufficient and a consistent time to meet as a team may be one of the biggest threats to a team's ability to carry out an effective program to address the social-communicative and behavior needs for students with ASD. As such, it will be of utmost importance to run meetings as efficiently as possible. Establishing team member roles described above, along with setting and adhering to specific ground rules will go a long way toward achieving efficiency; in addition, the following additional strategies discussed below are helpful.

Use of an Agenda

Have you ever attended a meeting and thought, "Why am I here?" Or, "What are we meeting for?" If so, odds are that an agenda was not made available during this meeting. Teams that utilize and adhere to a set meeting agenda achieve more than teams that do not. Agendas should include the primary objective(s) of the meeting, the roles that each team member will serve for that meeting, and a limited number (i.e., three to five) of discussion items with an allocated amount of time for each item indicated

(Table 6–3). Additionally, providing a brief time period at the beginning of the meeting to review the minutes from previous meetings, to add and/or remove items from the current meeting agenda, and to share successes and challenges is a good way to allow team members to informally engage prior to getting down to business. This may help to reduce off-topic sharing during discussion of specific agenda items. The agenda will be the common document that all team members will refer to as they assume their respective role during the meeting. The facilitator leads the team through each item, the timekeeper provides transition prompts based on the time allocated for each item, and the notetaker uses the agenda as the basis for recording minutes.

Action Planning

How many meetings have you attended where no follow-up activities or plans were agreed on or identified? Given that the entire purpose of meeting as a team is to enhance the effectiveness of programming and activities for students, it is essential that specific actions are identified and agreed to. To enhance the effectiveness of the team's activities, each team meeting should result in a written action plan outlining **what** specific activities will be achieved, **when** the team anticipates completing the activity, and **who** will take the lead on each activity. The Action Plan (Table 6–4) guides all of the team's activities in developing effective supports for students with ASD. As such, it should be a "living document." This means that the

Table 6–3. Sample Team Meeting Agenda

Team Meeting Agenda/Minutes		
Date:	Time:	Location:
Facilitator:	Timekeeper:	Participants:
Recorder:	Snackmaster:	
Next Facilitator:	Next Timekeeper:	Next Meeting Date, Time, and Location:
Next Recorder:	Next Snackmaster:	
Checking In		
Successes:		
Challenges:		
Items	**Action/Results**	
Review progress on action plan		
Persons, responsibilities, and timelines for next action plan activities		
Follow-up items from previous meeting		
Additional items		
Next steps/to do list:		

action plan should be present at each team meeting; time to review progress on the items on the plan should always be provided on the agenda, and the notetaker should update any revisions to a master version of the action plan. Although IEP teams will be able to use the IEP document itself as a sort of action plan, the type of action plan we are describing here can be used in the earliest developmental stages of team collaboration when putting together an

Table 6–4. Sample Team Action Planning Form

Team Action Plan				
Date:		Team Focus (Student/Committee Name):		
Team Members:				
Include information on the development, implementation, and monitoring activities of your plan for enhancing Social-Communication Skills for student(s) with ASD.				
Action Item/Activity (**What** will we do?)	Team Member Responsible (**Who** will take the lead?)	Start Date (**When** will we start?)	Completion Date (**When** will we finish?)	Is the Team Satisfied with the Results? (Yes/No)
1.				
2.				
3.				
4.				
5.				
6.				
7.				

IEP, and/or when focusing on a specific aspect of the IEP, such as when planning to teach social-communicative skills.

Distribution of Minutes

Have you ever left a meeting and immediately wondered, "What did I just agree to do?" Or rather, how many meetings have you attended nervously wondering, "Was I supposed to have accomplished something before this meeting?" A relatively simple yet essential component of effective collaboration involves sharing information that was discussed and agreements made during team meetings. In this current digital age, it has never been easier to share information with others. Rather than printing out or copying paper versions of meeting minutes and placing these in boxes in the school office and sending them home to parents, minutes can now easily be e-mailed to team members. Alternatively, many schools use cloud computing and/ or secure shared networks where documents, including meeting minutes, can easily be uploaded and accessed by team members at their convenience. Whatever the mechanism (low tech or high tech), the crucial consideration is to ensure that each team member receives a written documentation of agreements, decisions, action plans, responsibilities, and so forth, that were made during the meeting.

The Importance of Role Release

Although IDEA only requires a multidisciplinary team with members from multiple areas of expertise and responsibility to oversee the educational planning for students with disabilities, best practice suggests that teams should move beyond this approach toward a transdisciplinary teaming process for collaboration (Westling & Fox, 2009). A transdisciplinary teaming process is best characterized by a strategy referred to as "role release." Role release refers to the notion that no particular team member holds a monopoly on any particular area of expertise or role responsibility. Rather, team members are free, and in fact encouraged, to step outside of their traditional roles in order to take on and learn new skills and responsibilities. For example, the speech-language pathologist (SLP) should not be the only team member who contributes to the development of evidence-based strategies related to improving a student's social-communicative skills. Special and

general education teachers, classroom assistants, and family members should all be involved to ensure the contextual relevance and social validity of any communicative strategies to be implemented. They should also be involved in various aspects of this instruction to ensure generalization of skills across settings and social partners. Furthermore, under the guidance and support of the SLP, these team members may learn to take on additional roles traditionally reserved for the SLP. For example, the general education teacher may create a social narrative for teaching appropriate social-communicative skills during small group work in the general education classroom. A parent may learn to implement Pivotal Response Training at home or in the community to teach the student how to request preferred items appropriately. Additionally, a special education teacher may learn to create video models to teach social interactions with peers during an unstructured free time activity. In this scenario, the SLP might also engage in nontraditional activities. For example, the SLP might lead a brief lesson in the general education classroom, while the teacher reads the social story with the student. Alternatively, the SLP may lead students in the special education classroom through the lunch routine at the cafeteria, while the instructional assistant shows video clips to a student. In an effort to provide the best possible support to the student, the common theme in role release is to enhance collaboration so that team members have opportunities to expand their skills into new settings and activities. The HQC-A can support the teacher to recruit information from team members with regard to those areas in which they would like to expand their knowledge and expertise outside of their traditional roles. The Team Member Interest Inventory (Table 6–5) is a tool that can be used to collect this information and stimulate brainstorming around how best to provide these important opportunities for role release.

The vignette in Box 6–3 paints a common portrait of a small school district coming face-to-face with impending legal challenges and the implementation of services for children with ASD.

Table 6–5. Team Member Interest Survey

Team Member Interest Survey	
Date:	Team Focus (Student/Committee Name):
Team Member:	
In order to foster a true sense of collaboration, teams can support the development of new skills and experiences among their team members. This can allow for an increased ability to "share the load," and enhance one's own satisfaction with the team process. Please provide the information requested below. This will be shared at an upcoming team meeting to promote brainstorming with our collaborative efforts.	
1. What would you identify as your area of expertise (e.g., teaching, parenting, assessment, behavior support, knowledge of the student, etc.)?	
2. Skills or knowledge you would like to enhance *within* your area(s) of expertise. a. List the skills or knowledge you would like to obtain.	
2. Skills or knowledge you would like to enhance *within* your area(s) of expertise. b. List any activities that would assist you in learning these areas.	
3. Skills or knowledge you would like to enhance *outside of* your area(s) of expertise. a. List the skills or knowledge you would like to obtain.	
3. Skills or knowledge you would like to enhance *outside of* your area(s) of expertise. b. List any activities that would assist you in learning these areas.	

Box 6–3. Vignette: Catch Twenty-Two

Morgan is a first-grade student with mild symptoms of ASD who displays subtle deficits in social communication. One of his greatest challenges is peer acceptance. He has difficulty staying on topics that are of relevance to his peers' interests and often gives up on interactions with others in the classroom. When conversations fail, the district resource specialist has observed that Morgan may launch into repetitive verbal scripts about a narrow range of topics, which further alienates him from his classmates. Morgan loves the physical activity of swinging and is exceptionally skilled at upper body strength and control, but opportunities to practice his gross motor skills are often thwarted at recess. On the playground, he is unable to advocate for his turn on the climbing equipment, often being shoved aside as kids clamor to take control of the play equipment.

Morgan is included in a regular education program, where he is achieving at grade-level in all academic areas, but his parents are very concerned about his ability to make friends and defend himself from bullies. Parents are pleased with the general education teacher, but strongly object to allowing one member of the special education team to provide needed services to their son because they object to the traditional pull-out therapy model this provider uses; they refuse to sign the IEP, and instead, correspond with the district special education director about their objections, and propose that the district hire a different provider for these services. Parents have warned that they are close to filing for a legal hearing with a state-appointed administrative law judge to adjudicate the matter. The director of special education is eager to have the parents' consent to the pending IEP, although he is aware that his staff has minimal experience providing accommodations to students with ASD included in the general education setting. He is aware that the district's IEP offer will not be considered appropriate unless parents agree to necessary related services and supports that expressly address Morgan's major area of need: social communication. The director contacts the local educational agency for help. Parents are agreeable to having an autism consultant-coach meet with them, but have trepidation about going forward with the same provider. How can the program consultant help the district resolve this standoff before legal action becomes a reality?

The enigma is how to provide a defensible IEP for students' unique needs with staff who are underprepared for serving students like Morgan. Although there are no quick fixes to this situation, the district is aware of its obligation to provide services that are appropriate with respect to the Free and Appropriate Public Education, or FAPE standard. Even though school district capacity for doing so is presently limited, the intensive autism services coach and special education (SPED) administrator in this scenario join forces to craft initial solutions. Starting with common goal seeking (see Chapter 4), the consultant meets with the SPED administrator, and utilizing the list of steps (shown below in Table 6–6) establishes communication with the parents and members of the IEP team, including the district provider, to build common agreements as illustrated in Box 6–4.

Table 6–6. Solution-Finding Steps

1. Identify a few goals your team would like to work toward accomplishing.
2. Brainstorm ways that you think you can attain the goals your team has identified.
3. Winnow the goals down to one pressing immediate goal and an intermediate goal.
4. Organize materials or notes that team members may have already gathered to address the identified goals.
5. Discuss and write down any perceived barriers to reaching the stated goals.
6. After identifying perceived barriers, take time to clarify the goals.
7. Develop an action plan.
8. Develop a follow-along plan.
9. Evaluate progress toward reaching the stated goals.
10. Celebrate success.

Box 6–4. Case Study:
Morgan's Collaborative Teaming Process

In reference to the vignette "Catch Twenty-Two" and the Solution-Finding Steps (see Table 6–6), the information provided below illustrates the practical application of collaborative teaming processes applied to a real-world scenario with Morgan's Team.

- Meet, Brainstorm, and Identify Immediate and Intermediate Goals (Steps 1–3 in Table 6–6).
  - Following an initial meeting, the intensive coach, SPED Director, and parents of Morgan collaborated and arrived at two goals; one was immediate given the school year timeline as it was nearing the end of the school year and was specific to Morgan's unique Social Communication (SC) needs. This goal entailed collecting observations and recording Morgan's social interactions to familiarize the team with his unique SC profile and guiding the team to identify SC objectives based on his present levels of performance. The second goal was overarching in scope and long term: develop capacity of the faculty and staff to serve students in the school district with challenges similar to Morgan's.

- Organize Materials for Team to Identify the Goals (Step 4 in Table 6–6)
  - Discussion at the initial meeting ensued about how to implement the first goal. The district enlisted the coach to work with the IEP team; the coach provided materials for prioritizing Morgan's SC objectives (Step 4, Table 6–6), and shared intervention strategies that target those objectives. To address the second, long-term goal, the coach would provide professional development and follow-up training to faculty and SPED staff to improve their knowledge about the neurodevelopmental differences of children with ASDs and evidence-based interventions that target

the core deficits of children with this diagnosis (see Chapter 2).

- Identify Potential Barriers (Step 5 in Table 6–6)
    - In a separate meeting with the SPED director and case manager for Morgan, the following issues were identified as potential barriers for successful implementation of the goals.
    - Interpersonal barriers:
        - For the coach: Establishing trust with the district SPED team that, by all indications, was reluctant to accept coaching guidance. In a follow-up discussion with these providers, an objection was made that the SPED administrator had yielded to the parents' unreasonable demands.
        - For the coach: Building and establishing trust with the parents who want to be informed of steps put in place for improving outcomes for their son.
        - For the IEP Team: Repairing and reestablishing the relationship between provider and parents.
    - Resource barriers:
        - Availability of the coach, who is unable to be at the school site "24-7" to monitor classroom activities for implementing the SC objectives.

- Execute a Plan of Action (Step 7 in Table 6–6)
    - The following action plan was carried out:
        - Classroom Observation: Coach conducts an updated observation of Morgan in his classroom and in less-structured school settings (recess and lunch) to identify his core challenges as well as relative strengths in social communication. The coach records observational notes in the form described in Chapter 5 (see Table 5–3).
        - Follow-up Meeting: Coach shares observational findings with parents and the IEP team and proposes several SC objectives that target Morgan's greatest challenges. At this meeting,

coach and IEP team, along with Morgan's parents to prioritize three social communication (SC) objectives.

- Video Baseline: Coach conducts follow-up observation of Morgan in the classroom to collect a video baseline of his peer-to-peer interactions.

- Professional Development: Coach provides the IEP team and the general education teacher assigned for the upcoming year with an overview of Morgan's SC profile, sharing portions of the video of his peer social interactions, and brainstorming with others about embedding the three SC objectives in activities of the school day, including recess, lunch, and whole-school events (assemblies, recitals).

- IEP Meeting: SC goals are added to Morgan's addendum IEP document in addition to a report of his progress on his current IEP goals.

■ Develop a Follow-Along Plan (Step 8 in Table 6–6)

- Next Steps: Coach and IEP Team, including the parents, discuss a Team Action Plan to implement at the beginning of the school year (see Table 6–4). The plan was typed into a slide show and shared as a visual tool for the IEP Team.

Summary

This chapter explored the importance of building a team, identifying roles and responsibilities of its members, running efficient team meetings with planned agendas, and the advantages of engaging teams in role release. High-quality coaches ensure that team members collaborate effectively with one another. They can also empower the teacher to initiate collaboration and leadership of various constituencies in the classroom. The teacher's role is one of facilitator of a group of adults providing various supports to students. However, at times, particular individuals can supersede the teacher's role, which leads to inconsistent implementation and even conflict among adults in the classroom. When conflict is inevitable, the HQC-A plays a vital role in arriving at an action plan for resolving impasse. Coaching teachers on how to implement the techniques for effective collaboration and team functioning described in this chapter can set the foundation for successful implementation of effective programming to address the comprehensive needs of students with ASD.

plan for pursuing your own professional development activities as identified in the Team Member Interest Survey (see Table 6–5) in question #2.

End-of-Chapter Questions

1. From Table 6–1, select your personal top five tips for working with families. Provide a rationale for why each tip was selected.

2. Striving for mastery can be difficult when working with students with ASD. It requires patience, good instructional practice, and consistency. In this chapter we ask the coach to help a teacher with sending notes home to parents using a Daily Note Home form (see Table 6–2). This example is specifically geared for the teacher to master a daily parent-teacher communication process. Identify an area that you need to strive for mastery with respect to your communication with parents, or another skill area that needs attention. Remember to focus on you and your behavior. How would a coach be helpful in this situation?

3. Complete the Team Member Interest Survey (see Table 6–5) from this chapter. Share the results with a mentor, and discuss plans for your own professional development.

4. Use the Action Plan (see Table 6–4) of this chapter to develop an action

References

Crone, D. A., & Horner, R. H. (2003). *Building positive behavior support systems in schools: Functional behavior assessment.* New York, NY: Guilford.

Dunlap, G., Newton, J. S., Fox, L., Benito, N., & Vaughn, B. (2001). Family involvement in functional assessment and positive behavior support. *Focus on Autism and Other Developmental Disabilities, 16,* 215–221.

Kluth, P. (2009). *Autism checklist: A practical reference for parents and teachers.* San Francisco, CA: Jossey-Bass.

Kluth, P. (2010). *You're going to love this kid! Teaching students with autism in inclusive schools* (2nd ed.). New York, NY: Brookes.

McLaughlin, T. W., Denney, M. K., Snyder P. A., & Welsh, J. L. (2012). Behavior support interventions implemented by families of young children: Examination of contextual fit. *Journal of Positive Behavior Interventions, 14,* 87–97.

National Research Council. (2001). *Educating children with autism.* Washington, DC: National Academies Press.

Smith, T. E. C., Gartin, B. C., Murdick, N. L., & Hilton, A. (2006). *Families and children with special needs: Professional and family partnerships.* Upper Saddle River, NJ: Pearson.

Turnbull, A., Turnbull, H. R., Erwin, E. J., Soodak, L. C., & Shogren, K. A. (2011).

Families, professionals, and exceptionality: Positive outcomes through partnerships and trust (6th ed.). Upper Saddle River, NJ: Pearson.

Westling, D. L., & Fox, L. (2009). *Teaching students with severe disabilities* (4th ed.). Upper Saddle River, NJ: Prentice-Hall/ Merrill.

CHAPTER 7

Using High-Quality Coaching to Support the Assessment of Student Need and Instructional Planning

When you learn, teach. When you get, give.
—Maya Angelou

Chapter Objectives

- Provide coaches, teachers, and teams with a collaborative structure for approaching assessment of student need.

- Introduce key members of the team responsible for assessing student need.

- Justify using a variety of assessment strategies to unlock essential student skills.

- Provide teams and coaches with strategies for implementing informal assessment measures and baseline assessment for students with autism spectrum disorder (ASD).

- Describe examples of ecologically valid assessment of students with ASD.

Introduction

An important, but often overlooked, collaborative process for coaches and teachers is assessment planning to guide the selection of meaningful IEP goals and objectives. Assessment is necessary for establishing Individualized Education Program (IEP) goals and for informing progress monitoring about student academic achievement and functional performance, so it is crucial that teachers become familiar with a wide range of standardized and informal assessment tools to approach students' unique learning profiles. Teachers benefit from access to state-of-the art measurement tools and achieve insight into ways to conduct various assessments from high-quality coaches experienced in this area of practice. Research examining teacher preparation requirements for educating students with ASD has stressed the importance of the following: (a) conducting relevant assessment, (b) appropriately interpreting assessment results, and (c) matching assessment results to evidence-based educational decisions (Iovannone, Dunlap, Huber, & Kincaid, 2003; Yell, Drasgow, & Lowrey, 2005). Preservice instruction in this curricular area is the focus of university and college coursework for credentialing teachers in special education. Once teachers embark on their teaching careers, they must also learn how to approach assessment flexibly for it to become part of their professional repertoire (Yell et al., 2005). Ongoing assessment opens a window for teachers in evaluating their own instructional effectiveness over the course of the school year (Boutot & Smith Myles, 2010). A highly qualified coach specializing in ASD (HQC-A) recognizes the importance of this retrospective process, guiding teachers on how to make ongoing progress monitoring and probes of student performance a part of their core instructional approach.

High-quality coaching additionally helps pinpoint behavioral skills that need to be a focus for a student in managing the school day. Coaches and teachers provide a comprehensive picture of a student's strengths, weaknesses, motivation, and learning style from their classroom observations. Coaches can support this process by supplying information about how a student problem solves tasks, suspected barriers to learning, and specific resources for conducting specialized evaluation (e.g., providing tools designed to evaluate the core deficits of ASD in the areas of social communication and challenging behavior). Even though this information is useful for IEP report writing purposes as it encapsulates a student's overall present levels of performance, IEP goal writing is certainly the major objective of careful assessment planning. High-quality coaches help teachers achieve insight into ways to conduct relevant assessment so that IEP goals are embedded within naturally occurring events and classroom activities of the student's day. Consultative meetings with educational staff would also include suggestions by the coach about measurement tools having high validity. In particular, a high-quality coach directs the teacher to assessments that lead to the selection of meaningful instructional goals and effective strategies for instruction. Additional information will need to be obtained by the coach and addressed with the educational team given the unique resources and needs of each teacher and local school district. The HQC-A fulfills an instrumental role in working with the educational team to provide this information, and to seek out additional resources to support the assessment process. This chapter provides direction on many procedural components to this process.

Assessing for Student Need

As seen in the vignette in Box 7–1, instructional staff like Bea's general education teacher and inclusion assistant

---

Box 7–1. Vignette: Real Life

Halloween provided a learning experience for a teacher on how a young student with ASD handles zero structure. The kindergarten teacher provided her students with a very productive and healthy Halloween party. There were several activity centers set up: patterns, drawn-in details in scenery, making pizza, matching cards, and others. These centers were educational and fun. Students were asked to complete centers on their own time and had the choice of which centers to attend. Bea took the directions literally and only went to one center, the only one with stickers (she enjoys stickers). Parents were asked by the teacher not to pack snacks; snacks would be provided at school. Bea's inclusion support assistant relayed what happened next.

> I tried everything to get Bea to the snack centers. She doesn't like pizza and doesn't like apples. Bea was extremely over-stimulated by her costume and spent most of the day twirling and feeling her veil. The kindergarten teacher is awesome and made sure Bea was provided an alternative snack: a plain English muffin. Bea didn't eat a thing, and I barely got her to sit down. I used napkins to get her attention. First, I placed my napkin on the snack bench and sat down; I told her "this is how princesses sit." I then placed her napkin down and told her it was her turn, and then she sat down, but that was the only time she listened to me. Bea is a very sweet girl, so I was not too frustrated. The experience did educate me on how important assessing functioning within routines is for individuals with ASD.

have their hands full during the school day establishing and maintaining a class schedule, providing and creating materials for lessons, in addition to handling interruptions and challenging behaviors from students that can disrupt the flow of instruction, as well as managing the daily activity schedule. With these challenges before them, it is no surprise that teachers may err in targeting a student's essential needs. Teachers may follow a standardized test protocol to formally assess a student's skills when arriving at present levels of academic achievement and functional performance. However, since students with ASD often progress inconsistently in academic and in other core skill areas, particularly in social communication and appropriate prosocial behavior, assessment of their essential needs can seem gargantuan in scope, and zeroing in on their needs can be difficult. Some have a skill repertoire that is splintered with exceptionally high abilities in some areas, and deficits that swing to the other extreme. If the student is included in general education academic settings, what he or she can do in a given activity may not generalize as a mastered skill elsewhere in the school curriculum, or in a different classroom setting with typically developing peers. An effective HQC-A serving in a consultative or intensive coaching role has the benefit of evaluating such inconsistencies in skill sets, helping the teacher uncover student learning weaknesses, motivations, and preferences. Many students with ASD have difficulty understanding the relevance, or the "why," of what they are asked to learn. Consequently, their engagement

is limited in activities that lack natural motivation or are not developmentally sensible (Prizant, Wetherby, Rubin, Laurent, & Rydell, 2006). Moreover, without clearly defined structure in classrooms, students with ASD have immense challenges understanding what may happen next in the school day and predicting the sequences of events or steps within tasks so they can follow along. This was the case for Bea (see Box 7–1) as she failed to understand what the expectations were for the Halloween party. She simply could not adapt to the sudden departure from routine despite the best efforts and modeling by the instructional assistant.

Key Members of the Assessment Team

Because interdisciplinary assessment is regarded as best practice for evaluating individuals with ASD (NRC, 2001), the coach's role logically extends to working with multiple professionals of the educational team. Figure 7–1 identifies four critical members of the educational assessment team and their typical areas of assessment focus.

As emphasized elsewhere in this chapter, the teacher's role in assessment is critical for arriving at an overall summation of the student's present levels of achievement and functional performance. Preacademic assessment is necessary for preschool-aged children and for students who are developmentally less advanced yet acquiring the foundational skills that support literacy (read-

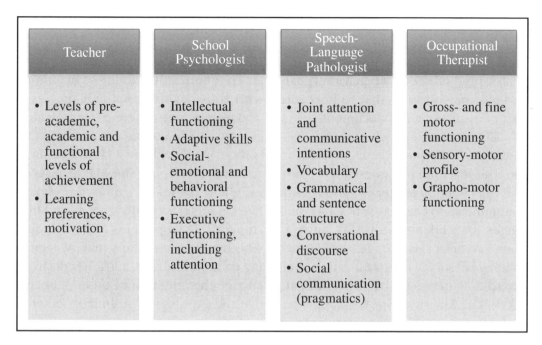

Teacher	School Psychologist	Speech-Language Pathologist	Occupational Therapist
• Levels of pre-academic, academic and functional levels of achievement • Learning preferences, motivation	• Intellectual functioning • Adaptive skills • Social-emotional and behavioral functioning • Executive functioning, including attention	• Joint attention and communicative intentions • Vocabulary • Grammatical and sentence structure • Conversational discourse • Social communication (pragmatics)	• Gross- and fine motor functioning • Sensory-motor profile • Grapho-motor functioning

Figure 7–1. Members of the assessment team and areas of assessment focus.

ing and written language) and math. There are multiple assessment measures designed to formally evaluate academic skills, including reading decoding, reading comprehension, spelling and written language, mathematical operations, and analysis. Assessment of functional skills that support an individual's daily living and independence in home and community settings is also the purview of the teacher. Above all else, the teacher's input to the assessment process about the student's learning style, his or her learning preferences, and unique motivation is of utmost value to the assessment team, including the HQC-A.

The school psychologist has primary responsibility for initially evaluating and updating the student's cognitive, adaptive, and behavioral and/or social-emotional status tri-annually as is re-

quired by law and as often as necessary to provide updated information about the student's intellectual, behavior, and social-emotional status. The latter skill domain is particularly important for older students with ASD, who often demonstrate "comorbid" psychiatric conditions influencing their regulatory behavior, attention, and executive functioning. For instance, anxiety and mood disorders are strikingly frequent in adolescents with ASD (Atwood, 2004; Simonoff et al., 2008) and impact a student's response to his or her environment, potentially leading to challenging behavior and resultant "meltdowns." In many specialized programs for students with ASD, educational agencies employ a qualified behavior specialist tasked with conducting functional assessment of the events that precede and follow challenging behavior. Instructional teams and families are especially reliant upon the detailed information provided by this analysis and subsequent behavioral goals and recommendations that will become part of a student's IEP document.

The school speech-language pathologist (SLP) plays a major role on the interdisciplinary assessment team. The SLP is knowledgeable about core communication characteristics and challenges for students with ASD, such as joint attention, language, and other aspects of social communication (see Kasari & Patterson, 2012; Prizant et al., 2006). The American Speech-Language-Hearing Association (ASHA) guidelines delineate the following communication areas when assessing students on the autism spectrum: (a) spontaneous initiation with various partners in a variety of social settings; (b) comprehension of verbal and nonverbal discourse in social, academic, and community settings; (c) the range of social functions engaged in by the student that are reciprocal and promote the development of friendships and social networks; and (d) verbal and nonverbal means of communication, including natural gestures, speech, signs, pictures, written words, as well as other alternative augmentative communication systems (ASHA, 2015).

The SLP's role on the assessment team is critical in differentiating between an ASD diagnosis and a "social communication disorder," a *Diagnostic and Statistical Manual of Mental Disorders* (5th edition) (*DSM-5*) diagnostic category involving impairment in the pragmatics of language without accompanying restricted or repetitive patterns of behavior (see Chapter 2). The SLP conducts formal and informal assessment of children who vary in their developmental communicative abilities, beginning with those at the prelinguistic stages of development, where communicative gestures, joint attention, and other nonverbal signals convey a child's communicative intentions. The SLP also lends insight to any idiosyncratic communicative strategies not fully understood by a student's social partners (e.g., a student who may scratch others may be signaling communicatively his or her desire to engage the attention of others). Receptive and expressive vocabulary, sentence and grammatical structure, conversational discourse skill (e.g., maintaining topic, making conversational repairs), and other social pragmatic skills are assessed by the SLP in individuals with advanced language use (Schoen Simmons, Paul, & Volkmar, 2014; Tager-Flusberg et al., 2009).

Most classrooms serving students with ASD have a school occupational therapist (OT) on the assessment team responsible for evaluating gross- and fine-motor skills, including graphomotor and adaptive fine-motor skills, such as buttoning and using zippers for dressing. The OT provides input to the educational team about how these skill areas impact the child's willingness to undertake demanding preacademic or academic tasks (e.g., cutting, pasting, copying, handwriting and written language). Importantly, evaluation is also undertaken of the child's sensory processing profile, which yields information about sensory preferences and avoidances. Motor and sensory-motor preferences and avoidances influence a child's self-confidence and personal reserves for coping with frustration. A child, for instance, who finds gripping and controlling a pencil difficult will be exceedingly challenged copying text, or generating lengthy amounts of text throughout the school day.

Formal Assessment

Even before the HQC-A conducts an initial observation of a classroom, one of the first steps of embedding assessment support is to get familiar with the student's presenting profile in a preobservation visit with the teacher and team. Members of the educational team and related therapy service providers should comprehensively undertake a process of "mining" available data about the student from work samples and records. Performance on formal, or standardized, assessments including psychoeducational evaluations and findings from other discipline reports is certainly one way to gain this insight. Typically, this includes the student's intellectual functioning, daily living and adaptive skills, fine and gross motor abilities, language and social communication skills, and academic levels of achievement. If not current, a teacher will want to update assessment of a student's preacademic, academic, and/or functional academic skills to share with the HQC-A. In the remaining sections of this chapter, we address other ways in which an HQC-A and educational teams can collaboratively problem solve student need utilizing a range of informal and baseline

assessment strategies that examine natural learning environments, or "milieus" (Roberts, Kaiser, Wolfe, Bryant, & Spidalieri, 2014).

Formal assessment information is comparative in nature. It generates a descriptive statistic, or set of scores, that provides an overview of where the student ranks relative to a similar population of peers, or normative group. In addition, assessment is often broadened to include less formal measures, because additional information is needed about a student's response style or, at the very least, suspected reasons for his or her behavioral responses that standardized assessment measures often overlook. If consideration has not also been given to nonstandardized assessments, the HQC-A can guide the teacher and assessment team in this direction utilizing a variety of criterion referenced tools, teacher-constructed probe tests, or other informational data gathering on the student. A teacher may also have curriculum and benchmark test scores, performance on screening measures that probe suspected deficit areas, in addition to a host of anecdotal observations about the student that she or he would like to share with the coach to paint a fuller profile of the student's competencies and challenges. There is a plethora of resources for evaluating present levels of functional performance and academic achievement that the coach and assessment team extract from available records, or plan on collecting by observation, parent or staff interview and direct evaluation of the student. This information along with feedback from family, home, and community service providers, who can attest to how the student transfers skills to unstructured environments in social and community-based settings, is critical for a comprehensive assessment protocol. A sampling of potential sources for identifying present levels of functioning is provided in Table 7–1.

Table 7–1. Sample Assessment Sources for Determining Student Present Levels

Sources of Present Levels of Functional Performance and Academic Achievement
• Standardized test scores (e.g., from psychoeducational or other assessments) • Annual state achievement test data • Placement test scores • Proficiency and/or benchmark tests • Curriculum-based measures: program data and mastery tests • Academic skills: error patterns, rate, accuracy • Teacher and parent rating scales of behavior, social communication, etc. • Skill inventories • Work samples • Attendance • Letter grades • Performance in class: participation, work completion, independence • Discipline and/or behavioral reports • Vocational interests or inventories • Preferred interests of student

Informal Assessment

Also called "performance assessment" (Boutot & Smith-Myles, 2010), informal evaluation methods are used in addition to, or in place of, standardized measures to help plan for instruction, and to arrive at a valid "ecological" profile of a student's strengths and weaknesses. Ecological validity refers to the relevance of the assessment in reflecting meaningful outcomes for the student in his or her natural learning milieu. The National Research Council (2001) emphasized that skills for young children with ASD must have ecological validity and be taught in functional daily routines in natural settings with multiple social partners. Because socialization opportunities with peers are part of a critical skill set for a preschool population, assessment must be comprehensively focused in this area with this age group. Given that standardized assessments may not be appropriate or meaningful with many students falling in the "difficult to test" category, the desired goal is to target essential skills that have immediate relevance to the educational curriculum. Table 7–2 lists a few types of informal assessment measures that coaches and teachers utilize when assessing for student need.

Although the list in Table 7–2 is not exhaustive, the goal is for the HQC-A to guide the team in exploring known resources for assessing the student as well as helping set up opportunities to evaluate additional skills that the team deems essential for success. Very often this task entails utilizing a variety of

Table 7–2. Types of Informal Assessment Measures

Measure	Description
Curriculum based	Skills acquired as measured by a specific curriculum
Criterion referenced	Skill attainment as it pertains to a specific criterion, such as age, grade, or learning standard (e.g., educational benchmark assessments)
Work samples	Products of student work (writing samples, drawings)
Ecological inventory	Evaluates the context in which complex skill use will be performed and instructional targets relative to a student's current performance
Task analysis	Performance level at various steps required to complete a complex task (e.g., washing laundry)
Portfolios	Student work products collected over time

informal assessment procedures, including teacher-constructed probes, criterion-based tests, and technological supports that augment or replace response requirements that tax a student (e.g., electronic tablet applications, speech-generating devices, and/or computer-assisted writing software). The goal is to more comprehensively analyze how the student problem solves, including preferred learning modalities that enhance engagement and success. This objective may also include an ecological assessment of learning and environmental supports considered most effective for accommodating a student's unique learning preferences (see Prizant et al., 2006). Although informal assessment measures do not generate comparison scores about performance relative to a group standard or norm (e.g., typically developing peers of comparable chronological or mental age), a dis-

tinct advantage is the degree to which they evaluate a curriculum area, a particular developmental subskill, and/or level of skill mastery (Boutot & Smith Myles, 2010). As further illustrated by the vignette in Box 7–2, informal assessment is appropriate for targeting meaningful instructional goals and objectives and linking these to practical and effective teaching strategies in the classroom.

Informal procedures that press for the student's maximal learning potential are often regarded as "dynamic assessment" (Boutot & Smith-Myles, 2010). Dynamic assessment examines the most effective way to teach a particular skill via a specific learning modality (e.g., visual-spatial, auditory-verbal) utilizing teaching strategies that have the greatest impact by tapping into a student's learning strengths or preferences. Dynamic assessment examines learned skills in addition to emerging skills in a student's

---

Box 7–2. Vignette: Helping Jenny Read

Jenny showed up in my class as a student with ASD on an administrative placement from a neighboring school district. Although she is 9 years old, she is beginning to read with some degree of proficiency. However, the teacher is unable to discern how fluently she reads and whether or not she comprehends what she has read. The teacher had heard about curriculum-based measurement in her credential courses but thought it was more useful for students with learning disabilities. In an initial assessment, the teacher noticed that Jenny is able to read words across a page by putting her finger on the words and reading them one by one. After reading a couple of basic sentences, the teacher asked her what she had read. Jenny was only able to identify the character of the story but none of the content. The teacher decided that increasing Jenny's fluency would be a good place to start so that she would begin to coordinate scanning text across the page and read more fluidly. The teacher decided to have Jenny place a ruler under each sentence and then continue to have her point to each word. In addition, the teacher decided to access a curriculum-based reading assessment and provide 1-minute trials for Jenny with the hopes of increasing her reading fluency that would then improve comprehension. The teacher contacted her HQC-A assigned from the district to work with her so she could brainstorm about the curriculum-based strategy she was thinking of employing.

---

repertoire and contextual supports that maximize response success (ASHA, 2015). Also referred to as "diagnostic teaching," this type of assessment can be extremely useful for an HQC-A taking observational notes on how the student responds to teacher/examiner feedback, and for translating student-teacher interactions during a test-teach process (see Boutot & Smith Myles, 2010).

Another informal assessment tool is the ecological inventory, and/or task analysis procedure like the one displayed in Table 7–3. The advantage of ecological inventories is that they examine students in natural settings, often in spontaneous communicative exchanges. Ecologically valid measures inform the teacher and educational team about skill generalization. Task analyses break down

Table 7–3. Sample Ecological Inventory for Communication Skills

Domain: Communication

Environment: Elementary School

Sub-Environment: Playground

Skill: Responding to greetings from others

Task Analysis:

1. Stop engaging in current activity
2. Orient face toward the communicative partner
3. Make eye contact with partner
4. Say "hi," "hello," "wanna play?"
5. Resume activity and take turns with peer at an activity

a larger skill into manageable steps that make instruction systematic. This type of informal analysis relates directly to the subskills needed by the student to be successful in typical classroom and community activities and routines. A useful task analysis for an older student may entail the steps for washing and drying clothing in a community Laundromat.

In the area of social communication and pragmatics (i.e., the rules that govern language use in social contexts; Bates, 1979), it is important that the assessment team and coach explore social communicative contexts in which students, including those with advanced language skills, typically struggle. Direct observation in unstructured interactions with peer and adult partners is the most ecologically valid means for undertaking this objective. Table 7–4 provides examples of several informal measures as-

sessing a student's social communication profile. Each measure differs in its construction, explicit purpose, and target age group or age range. The list consists of parent and teacher/clinician rating scales and dynamic observational tools useful for evaluating social communication skills that otherwise may be missed in fast-paced social exchanges.

Informal assessment methods are ideal for discovering the conceptual processes used by a learner to arrive at a given response (Boutot & Smith Myles, 2010). The teacher's focus is on interpreting *how the student interacts with his or her learning environment* relative to observable behaviors (e.g., frustration tolerance, self-correction of errors, and evidence of problem-solving strategies). Examiner corrective feedback, for example, offered when the student responds inaccurately to test items, is useful to explore the limits of a student's problem solving. Another informal evaluation strategy is recording student behavior and response patterns when change-of-task requirements are introduced. Teachers and observing coaches should notice how the student responds when aspects of the learning task, including the presentation mode (e.g., auditory-verbal, visual, tactile) are systematically manipulated. Providing a visual support during a writing assessment such as a word web, or other visual graphic organizer can help a student having difficulty comprehending written language instructions, enhance organization of written content, and provide a picture of how well the student utilizes strategic instructional supports.

Table 7–4. Sample Assessment Measures of Social Communication

Test Name	Author(s)	Publication Date	Description	Applicable Age Range
Children's Communication Checklist	Bishop	2006	Parent/Caregiver rating scale of pragmatic and conversational skills	4 to16 years
Language Use Inventory	O'Neil	2009	Standardized observational measure of speech acts and communicative functions	18 to 47 months
McArthur–Bates Communicative Development Inventory	Fenson et al.	2006	Standardized parent/ caregiver inventory of first communicative gestures, words, and sentences	8 to 30 months
Targeted Observation of Pragmatics in Children's Conversation	Adams et al.	2012	Semistructured observational rating of basic conversational skills; picture supported	6 to 11 years
Treatment and Research Institute for ASDs–TRIAD (2nd ed.)	Stone et al.	2010	Criterion referenced. Parent, teacher rating scales and structured interactions (picture supported) to assess comprehension of emotions, perspective taking, social initiation, and social maintenance	6- to12- year-olds with basic reading skills
Yale *in Vivo* Pragmatic Protocol	Schoen Simmons et al.	2014	Semistructured assessment of conversational skill: discourse management, communicative functions, conversational repairs, and presuppositions	School age

Baseline Assessment

The concept of establishing a "baseline" evaluation of a student's skills prior to instructional support is equally impor- tant for establishing preinstructional assessment information useful for prog- ress monitoring of an IEP goal area. Baseline reflects some aspect of the student's overall present levels of performance in a specific skill area. Observable responses produced by the student are recorded *before* instruction or intervention is begun. Typically, some form of standardized assessment is conducted to hone in on deficit areas, and initial baseline data can then be collected on targeted skills in the IEP. The details of collecting baseline (and progress monitoring) data are described more extensively in Chapter 8.

Consultative Coaching Example

This section provides an example of how a coach might support a teacher in the assessment process using a consultative model based on the vignette in Box 7–3, "Unlocking Antonio." As described in this vignette, Antonio is a fairly high-functioning student with strengths in academics. His known weaknesses are socialization and self- advocacy, competencies that will have significant impact for his success at school and in his community. Antonio's educational team needs direction from the consultative coach about what to target as well as suggestions for assessment measures, both formal and informal, that will guide instructional planning.

The coach conducted an observation of Antonio, met with his team to review his assessment records, and conferred with the teacher and instructional assistant on additional informal assessments that would supply needed information about Antonio's social skills. A social rating scale was suggested to dynamically evaluate Antonio's social communication skills in natural settings,

---

Box 7–3. Vignette: Unlocking Antonio

As a one-to-one instructional assistant working with Antonio, a high school student with ASD, I have begun to understand the importance of my role in not only supporting Antonio, but ensuring he successfully integrates in mainstream content classes. Intellectually Antonio can handle the academic content with my assistance. He does have difficulty processing information and frequently engages in repetitive motor movements (tapping, waving his finger, and moving his legs up and down) when he stresses out. He also has trouble working with other students in pairs, triads, and cooperative learning groups. I have been instrumental in helping him join together with his peers and start to develop interpersonal skills that make him feel included and valued. None of what I do is done in a vacuum; I am in constant contact with Antonio's resource instruction specialist, the general education teachers, and Antonio's parents. We work as a team and consult continuously about his progress and successes at school. Here are a few of my thoughts.

Working with Antonio, who is included in general education classrooms, has been a great experience for me. It is amazing to observe and learn new things about him everyday. Not only is he learning in the classroom, but I am learning many new things myself as well. Multimedia is one of his favorite classes and, as a result, I began fading my support from this class because he does not need my support like he does in the other classes. Although today was different, he asked me to stay with him in the classroom so I could view one of the projects he was putting together. It is amazing to see how much talent this student has, and how much interest he takes in this class. He enjoys trains and discussing how trains move and are put together. Antonio is able to join in class activities and create things he never thought possible. I am excited to see what he will create in this classroom in the weeks to come.

Socialization is key for Antonio. In order for him to become successful in the classroom he is going to need to learn better peer interaction and social communication skills. He is uncomfortable asking his partner in the classroom, or asking his group in the class for help. Being able to step back and help him become more dependent on himself rather than dependent on me is also important. He is able to ask me for help, but he has a hard time processing all of the information that goes on in the classroom. It is my job to make sure he was able to learn all that. I am very curious to learn new ways to assess and help him develop skills to become independent. School is important for Antonio, and he understands that in order to be successful, 100 percent of his work needs to be done. He is capable of doing so much, and I have actually set up a few socialization goals (initiating and turn-taking with peers; changing topics appropriately when there are partner changes in agenda). I need to learn how to assess progress toward meeting those goals and to make sure I know what I am doing. I do not want to assume he should be doing more without assessing progress toward these goals.

and to compare ratings about his social competency from both teacher and parent. An informal social skills rating scale designed for students with ASD (e.g., Stone et al., 2010) was utilized for this purpose. In follow-up consultation with the educational team and family, the consultative coach helped team members link their assessment findings to clarify meaningful goals and objectives that targeted Antonio's identified weaknesses in social communication. Team members collectively decided on two essential skills: (a) initiating social activities with peers, and (b) independently asking for help to complete assignments. The HQC-A further guided the team to implement a baseline assessment of each of these goal behaviors to get an *initial* picture of Antonio's rate of peer social initiation, as well as the frequency of how often he initiated requests for help, either with instructional staff and/or with peer partners. The instructional assistant was instrumental in undertaking this data collection process over two to three consecutive school days so that teachers and staff had a clear idea of Antonio's current levels of initiations and requests for help. Baseline data helped the team make informed instructional decisions about *where* to conduct ecological inventories and task analyses of activities in which social initiations and requests for help would be expected to occur, and subsequently how to engineer the social environment for Antonio so he could be successful. Description of procedures for data collection methods, including task analytic data collection is detailed further in Chapter 8.

Intensive Coaching Example

In this section, an example of how the HQC-A could implement an intensive coaching model to support a teacher with the assessment process is described for Jason, a 7-year-old student with moderate-to-severe ASD and emerging verbal language skills. Jason had recently transferred from a local school district to a comprehensive special day program for students with ASD. Upon his arrival, his educational team felt obliged to continue his previous IEP goals as his previous team and parents had forged them over many hours of IEP meetings. However, it was soon apparent that a math goal addressing Jason's ability to recognize number symbols and corresponding quantities up to 15 was targeted well above his current level of functioning. Not only did Jason respond randomly to explicit training trials administered by the teacher who used number symbol cards and quantities, Jason became extremely agitated during instruction, grabbing materials and persistently biting his hand. The HQC-A noticed that when the teacher placed Jason at a kidney-shaped table pushed up against a wall so that he could not physically escape the task, his behavior worsened.

Jason's social communication initiations at school were minimal to non-existent. He was disengaged from peers, and it was evident that he did not interact socially with adults. This was noticeable during highly routine activities of the school day that specifically attempted to elicit his engagement (e.g., calendar time, art, and snack). His instructional assistant dutifully led him through activities of the day, but it was apparent to the HQC-A that Jason did not engage in any spontaneous turn-taking with partners in these activities. Although the teacher and IEP team were confused about what direction to take with Jason, the coach helped develop an action plan similar to the one discussed for intensive coaching in Chapter 5 using the Team Action Planning Form found in Chapter 6 (Table 6–4). A completed form appears in Table 7–5 identifying team members, team responsibilities, and agreed upon timelines. The process for undertaking this coaching experience was intensive. The HQC-A began by recording a video clip of Jason during the school day, sharing segments of the video with the team so that they could (a) objectively evaluate his challenges, (b) collectively decide on a practical way to evaluate Jason's math levels, and (c) construct new social communication goals addressing his primary difficulty with social participation.

With intensive coaching support, the math goal was revised to align with Jason's current skill levels and his present ability to demonstrate an understanding of the concept of "one" versus "more than one." Additionally, a new social communication goal was prioritized for increasing his engagement in daily activities introduced as part of the school curriculum. The goal was implemented by engaging Jason in reciprocal turn-taking exchanges during sensory-motor and gross-motor activities that were highly motivating and preferred (e.g., blowing bubbles at circle time,

using colorful art materials at a table-top, and in back-and-forth exchanges with playground equipment during his OT therapy).

Jason made improvement in his spontaneous interactions with staff, but along the way he also displayed behaviors that were challenging for the team to deal with. These consisted of biting adults and children and bolting from the classroom. His family was understandably alarmed and requested extended meetings with the teacher and behavior specialist. Disagreements on how best to proceed wore down team morale. Hence, an important step of the coaching process in this case involved regular follow-up by the HQC-A with the team to instill confidence and a sense of competence when working with Jason. In this intensive delivery model, the HQC-A reviewed video clips of Jason's engagement in school activities over multiple weeks to share documented successes with both the team and the family. Team meetings were constructed in the same format as discussed in Chapter 6, where each participant at the meeting had a role to fulfill (e.g., time keeping was particularly important so that meetings did not run exceedingly long). Over time, the coach tapered more intensive support with check-in times with the team. Prior to a Supplemental IEP meeting with the family, the coach met with the team to review Jason's social interactions at school and his functional performance on the math goal. Several positive assessment outcomes were evident from the original baseline video. Jason began to show enjoyment at school and,

Table 7–5. Action Planning Worksheet for Coaches and Teachers

Action Plan Worksheet: Jason

From Vision to Action

Today's Date: September 20

Purpose of Action Plan: Conduct observation, assessment and follow-up supplemental IEP meeting to revise IEP goals (math, social skills)

WHO	Will do WHAT	By WHEN/Status
HQC-A	a) Meet with teacher, team, and family to review available resources about student need: IEP documents, prior assessments, discipline reports, work samples, etc.	a) September 20
	b) Videotape math lesson in classroom activities of the day	b) October 20
School psychologist	Reassess intellectual and adaptive skills	October 30
SLP	Share language and social communication profiles with assessment team and family	September 20
Teacher	Construct informal instructional probes; assess comprehension of "more" versus "one" using preferred snack items/toys	September 30
OT	Share assessment findings of fine- and gross-motor preferences and skills with assessment team and family	September 20
HQC-A, teacher and assessment team	Meet with team; review baseline video of math lesson and Jason's classroom day; guide prioritization of IEP goals	October 30
HQC-A and Assessment Team + family	IEP Supplemental Meeting: review updated assessment findings and baseline video; reach consensus on two new goals	November 10

for the first time, engaged in sustained social initiation establishing "joint attention" and shared turn-taking with adult partners in the classroom. He began to show progress on his revised math goal responding accurately to activities where he could select more than one food item at snack, or request "more than one" preferred object or activity (e.g., asking for additional puzzle pieces and parts of cause-and-effect toys).

Summary

This chapter addressed high-quality coaching and assessment of students with ASD. A skilled HQC-A directs the educational team to be comprehensive in accessing all existing data about the student, and guides the assessment team to select appropriate measurement tools that examine the core deficits of ASD. The coach also supports the teacher and team with accurate interpretation of assessment findings, including behavior, to arrive at a summation of the student's levels of performance, academic achievement, and unique learning strengths and preferences. A range of formal and informal assessment tools is often necessary to identify and target essential skills. It is critical that a careful review of assessment outcomes from an interdisciplinary team of assessment specialists be undertaken, as each assessment specialist examines different skills areas of the student crucial to a full understanding of strengths and core challenges.

Informal assessment and baseline data collection reveal task demands and the relevance of IEP goals to be targeted, and the best means of approaching instruction. When teachers learn to regularly evaluate student progress to inform their classroom practices, the research-to-practice gap between teacher training and implementation of evidence-based educational practices can be minimized.

This increases the likelihood that interventions known to improve outcomes for students with ASD will be implemented with fidelity. HQC-A coaches lead the educational team to consider new and revised IEP goals, specialized assessments, and a full complement of evidence-based strategies, including classroom (environmental) and learning supports to implement assessment findings.

End-of-Chapter Questions

1. Assume you are the HQC-A for a middle school classroom of students with ASD. The teacher has indicated that he needs to write new IEP goals for a particular student, and that he has four IEP meetings scheduled in the next 6 weeks of instruction. Although the student has been previously and comprehensively evaluated, he is failing his inclusion language arts class and has several social challenges with peers (e.g., refuses to join cooperative groups and will not socially initiate with peers). What areas of additional assessment would you help guide the teacher and team to pursue? What members of the assessment team would you approach to undertake additional assessment?

2. List several informal assessment measures and/or strategies you have implemented as coach, instructor, or instructional assistant serving students with ASD. What additional insight did they contribute in your

determination of the students' present levels of academic achievement and functional performance?

3. Suggest some practical strategies that you have employed, or that you predict might be useful with a "difficult-to-assess" student.

4. Why is baseline assessment important? Discuss what additional assessment information a baseline provides beyond a battery of standardized academic tests.

5. Lee is a 10-year-old with high-functioning ASD with reading and receptive-expressive language skills that are grade appropriate. However, he detests any activities that call on him to write about what he has read. He is capable of written output but lacks motivation to complete assignments. As the HQC-A working with Lee's educational team, how will you help his team approach this challenge?

References

Adams, C., Lockton, E., Freed, J., Gaile, J., Earl, G., McBean, K., & Law, J. (2012). The social communication intervention project: A randomized controlled trial of the effectiveness of speech and language therapy for school-age children who have pragmatic and social communication problems with or without autism spectrum disorder. *International Journal of Language and Communication Disorders, 43*, 233–244.

American Psychiatric Association. (2013). *Diagnostic and statistical manual of mental disorders* (5th ed.). Washington, DC: Author.

American Speech-Language-Hearing Association. (2015). *Autism spectrum disorder: Assessment/diagnosis/screening*. Retrieved July 29, 2015, from: http://www.asha.org/PRPSpecificTopic.aspx?folderid=8589935303&section=Assessment

Atwood, T. (2004). Cognitive behaviour therapy for children and adults with Asperger's syndrome. *Behaviour Change, 21*(3), 147–161.

Bates, E. (1979). *The emergence of symbols: Cognition and communication in infancy*. New York, NY: Academic Press.

Bishop, D. (2006). *Children's communication checklist* (2nd ed.). London, UK: Psychological Corporation.

Boutot, E. A., & Smith Myles, B. (2010). *Autism spectrum disorders: Foundations, characteristics, and effective strategies*. New York, NY: Pearson.

Fenson, L., Marchman, V. A., Tahl, D. J., Dale, P. S., Reznick, J. S., & Bates, E. (2006). *The McArthur-Bates Communicative Inventory* (2nd ed.). Baltimore, MD: Brookes.

Iovannone, R., Dunlap, G., Huber, H., & Kincaid, D. (2003). Effects of educational practices for students with autism spectrum disorder. *Focus on Autism and Other Developmental Disabilities, 18*, 150–165.

Kasari, C. & Patterson, S. (2012). Interventions addressing social impairment in autism. *Current Psychiatry Reports, 14*(6), 713–725.

Laurent, A. C., & Rubin, E. (2004). Emotional regulation challenges in Asperger's syndrome and high functioning autism. *Topics in Language Disorders, 24*(4), 286–297.

National Research Council. (2001). *Educating children with autism*. Washington, DC: National Academy Press.

Prizant, B. M., Wetherby, A. M., Rubin, E., Laurent, A. M., & Rydell, P. J. (2006). *The*

SCERTS Model Program Planning and Intervention: A comprehensive educational approach for young children with autism spectrum disorders. Volume 2: Program planning and intervention. Baltimore, MD: Brookes.

Roberts, M. Y., Kaiser, A. P., Wolfe, C. E., Bryant, J. D., & Spidalieri, A. M. (2014). Effects of the teach-model-coach-review instructional approach on caregiver use of language support strategies and children's expressive language skills. *Journal of Speech, Language and Hearing Research, 57,* 1851–1869.

Schoen Simmons, E., Paul, R., & Volkmar, F. (2014). Assessing pragmatic language in autism spectrum disorder: The Yale in vivo pragmatic protocol. *Journal of Speech, Language, and Hearing Research, 57,* 2162–2173.

Simonoff, E., Pickles, A., Charman, T., Chandler, S., Loucas, T., & Baird, G. (2008). Psychiatric disorders in children with autism spectrum disorders: Prevalence, comorbidity, and associated factors in a population-derived sample. *Journal of the American Academy of Child and Adolescent Psychiatry, 47*(8), 921–929.

Stone, W., Ruble, L., Coonrod, E., Hepburn, S., Pennington, M., Burnette, C., & Bainbridge Brigham, N. (2010). *TRIAD Social Skills Assessment* (2nd ed.). Nashville, TN: Treatment and Research Institute for Autism Spectrum Disorders (TRIAD), Vanderbilt Kennedy Center.

Tager-Flusberg, H., Rogers, S., Cooper, J., Landa, R., Lord, C., Paul, R., . . . Yoder, P. (2009). Defining spoken language benchmarks and selecting measures of expressive language development for young children with Autism spectrum disorders. *Journal of Speech, Language, and Hearing Research, 52,* 643–652.

Yell, M. L., Drasgow, E., & Lowrey, K. A. (2005). No Child Left Behind and students with autism spectrum disorders. *Focus on Autism and Other Developmental Disabilities, 20,* 130–139.

CHAPTER 8

Using High-Quality Coaching to Support the Selection of Skills for Instruction and Monitoring Student Progress

No work is insignificant. All labor that uplifts humanity has dignity and importance and should be undertaken with painstaking excellence.

—Martin Luther King, Jr.

Chapter Objectives

■ Assist coaches and teachers in selecting skills for instruction.

■ Provide resources and strategies for the efficient collection of data on student progress.

Introduction

Ensuring that effective instruction is provided in meaningful ways to students with autism spectrum disorder (ASD) may be the most critical area in which coaches can support teachers. There are multiple areas in which coaches can focus their support to teachers when it comes to providing meaningful instruction. Coaches can support teachers in selecting skills to teach, defining skills to teach, developing efficient systems for tracking the use of skills selected, setting goals for skill development, selecting and delivering evidence-based strategies to teach selected skills, and analyzing data collected to ensure that progress is being made and/or revising instruction to maximize success. Each of these critical areas will be discussed below, with an emphasis on the collaborative role between the coach and the teacher in achieving effective instructional outcomes.

Selecting and Defining Skills to Teach (Where to Start?)

When integrating the results of assessments into the writing of goals and selection of instructional strategies, high-quality coaching–autism (HQC-A) coaches and teachers should keep some key principles in mind. These principles include (a) selecting and teaching *functional* skills, (b) promoting student *independence*, (c) ensuring that targeted skills are *meaningful*, (d) selecting skills that are *linked to student needs and*

strengths, and (e) ensuring that targeted skills are *operationally defined*. Adhering to these guiding principles will maximize not only the success of the student, but that of their family members and the collaborative team as well.

First, any skills selected should be *functional* to the everyday needs of the student. The term *functional* refers to the extent to which the skill is needed in order for the student to be successful in his or her natural environment: home, school, and community. Lou Brown, Nietupski, and Hamre Nietupski (1976) originally identified this principle as the Criterion of Ultimate Functioning, whereby the skills selected for instruction should be those that would benefit the individual in the future (i.e., his or her ultimate functioning). Ensuring that the skills we teach are those that the individual will use over the course of his or her life frees teachers from the "readiness trap," the idea that students need to "develop" further (typically without formal instruction to do so) before certain skills can be taught. Hence, considering the chronological age appropriateness of the skill to be taught directly impacts how functional a skill will be. When selecting a skill for instruction, the team should always ask, "How will this skill benefit the student in their day to day life?"

Relatedly, the skills targeted for instruction should promote the *independence* of the student. If the skills are intended to be used in everyday settings, then they should also be taught in a way so as to be used as independently as possible. To achieve independence, students will ultimately need to perform the skill in new settings, with different people, and when presented with new materials. Instructional strategies should be selected which promote the generalization of new skills from the outset. Additionally, the skill will need to be performed in the absence, or at least with the reduction of, instructional supports. Therefore, if additional prompts and contrived reinforcers are used to teach initial skill acquisition, clear plans and timelines will need to be developed indicating how these strategies will be faded out or reduced over time.

Not only should skills be functional and promote independence, but they should also be *meaningful* to those who will be directly impacted by their use. The person most impacted, of course, is the student. Therefore, it is critical to select "pivotal" skills for instruction. Pivotal skills are defined as those that when acquired result in response generalization, or improvements in other nontargeted skills (Koegel, Koegel, Harrower, & Carter, 1999). Given the often high number of skills that students with ASD will need to master in order to enhance outcomes, coaches and teachers need to teach these skills in the most efficient manner possible. Thus, targeting areas like student motivation, responsivity to multiple stimulus components, self-management, and self-initiations, such as question asking, can maximize the progress that students can make in acquiring new and meaningful skills. Additionally, to the greatest extent possible, the needs, preferences, and expressed desires of the student should be incorporated into the skill selection process by the team. The notion that the more an individual is involved in selecting the skills they will be taught, mak-

ing their own choices, setting their own goals, and advocating for themselves has been referred to as Self-Determination (Wehmeyer, Field, Doren, Jones, & Mason, 2004). A related concept that informs us as to whether or not a skill is meaningful is that of quality of life. Quality of life refers to the extent to which valued outcomes are available through typically available resources to the individual (Schalock, 2004). The key questions for the team in this area would be, "Is the skill important from the perspective of the student?" and "Will the skill be taught in a way that the student would prefer?" It is important to note, however, that the student is not the only person who stands to find skill development meaningful. Parents, siblings, and other family members also have a vested interest in which skills will be selected and taught, as the student's enhanced use of these skills can impact the quality of their lives as well. Thus, teams should actively engage both the student and his or her family in the selection of skills to teach.

Another important consideration when selecting skills to teach is that they should be *linked to student needs and strengths*. After reading the information presented in Chapter 7, this principle may seem obvious; however, after discussing the above principles of functional, meaningful, independent skill use, the team may need to revisit the assessment plan to ensure that the student's needs and strengths in these areas have been adequately assessed. Furthermore, if it appears that the available assessment results do not speak to these principles, coaches will want to provide support to the teacher in working with the team to select and administer additional assessments intended to capture this important information.

Once a set of instructional skills has been selected by the team, it is critical that they be *operationally defined*. An operational definition is one that is observable and measurable. When skills are defined operationally, they can be more effectively taught, and data collection systems can subsequently be developed to track student progress in their use of the skill(s). For example, rather than defining a skill as "Student will transition well in class," potentially meeting the functional/independent/meaningful principles, a more operational definition could be "When prompted, student will

walk quietly with all necessary materials to the next activity." Further, a definition such as this could be updated over time to illustrate how prompts will be faded in order to promote independence; for example, tracking of student transitions in the absence of prompts. Thus, prior to moving forward, teams should reach consensus on how the skill(s) will be operationally defined. Coaches can support teachers in this area by providing examples of operationally defined skills as well as feedback on how skills are initially defined.

Coaches and teachers can make use of the Team Checklist for Skill Selection available in Table 8–1 when working with the team to reach consensus on the

Table 8–1. Team Checklist for Skill Selection

Student Name				
Date				
Team Members Present				
Ratings	1 = No, 2 = Somewhat, 3 = Yes			
Criteria/Skills	Skill 1:	Skill 2:	Skill 3:	Skill 4:
Functional	1 2 3	1 2 3	1 2 3	1 2 3
Promotes Independence	1 2 3	1 2 3	1 2 3	1 2 3
Meaningful	1 2 3	1 2 3	1 2 3	1 2 3
Linked to Needs/Strengths	1 2 3	1 2 3	1 2 3	1 2 3
Operationally Defined	1 2 3	1 2 3	1 2 3	1 2 3
Overall Priority Score (out of 15):	/15	/15	/15	/15

whether the skills under consideration are functional, promote independence, are meaningful, and are operationally defined.

Measuring Skills (To What Extent Can the Student Perform the Skill?)

A key issue in providing effective instruction is to ensure that the team is fully aware of how the student is performing the skill over time, and in response to any interventions implemented. The use of data to inform instruction is a hallmark of evidence-based practice for students with ASD (National Standards Project, 2009). Collecting data on student performance allows the team to identify whether intervention is warranted, what type of intervention should be used, when skill development is not occurring and interventions need to be changed, and when skills have been mastered and intervention can be focused to promote generalization, faded out and/or terminated. However, as illustrated by the vignette in Box 8–1, these questions should guide the selection and use of data collection methods (rather than vice versa), and thus data collection should play an integral role in informing instructional decision making. A data collection system should be put in place by the team until it is designed to directly inform the way one would teach. Data collection is critical to effective instruction, yet data collection for data's sake (without a clear link back to instruction) is not

evidence-based practice. A primary role for coaches with regard to supporting teachers in the appropriate use of data collection will be to share and assist in the development of user-friendly data collection forms and methods. Multiple data collection methods are available to coaches and teachers for selection. We briefly discuss some of the more common methods used when designing appropriate data collection systems for students with ASD. These consist of Frequency, Interval, Latency, Duration, Task Analytic, and Trials to Criterion methods.

Frequency Data Collection Methods

Perhaps the most straightforward method for collecting data is to simply count the number of times a behavior or skill occurs. As seen in Table 8–2, tallying the number of times a student displays a targeted skill within a given period of time can be a quick and easy way to gain information on how the student is progressing in response to the instruction. However, there are limitations to this approach. First, skills that vary in the length of time displayed may not best be captured with a frequency data collection method. For example, tracking the frequency of interactions with peers may be insufficient in capturing the length and quality of the interactions, which may actually decrease in frequency as the duration increases over time. Second, certain skills may not have a clear start and a clear end, a requirement for frequency data collection. If a student is learning to perform multistep

Box 8–1. Vignette: Coaching Inside the Lines

Mrs. Tracy's child, Eddie, is a student at Myers Briggs Elementary School. He has been at the school since second grade and is now going into fifth grade. Mrs. Tracy is on Site Council, PTA, and a local disability parent network. She is well known for her advocacy on behalf of students with ASD. She attends state and national conferences bringing back the latest information on ASD. After she attends these conferences, she has a tendency to want the school to immediately incorporate these ideas in the classroom. Last month she attended the state conference on autism spectrum disorder and was introduced to Drs. Langsforth and Newsome, who are using a new technique known as STAR for Systematic Tracking and Rating, wherein the teacher records with a handheld clicker student initiations and responses in established 15-minute trial periods throughout the day. There must be nine trial periods per day, six in the morning and three in the afternoon. If the teacher misses one trial period, this must be noted and made up somewhere in the day or the next day. Make-ups have to be done that day or the next, or the data, according to the researchers, are invalid. Mrs. Tracy is on board with this new method believing this as the next great breakthrough in teaching children with ASD. Though she is well respected at school and throughout the school district, the teachers, and support staff are not willing to endorse this method. Their response to Mrs. Tracy is diplomatic, indicating that they have a very rigorous behaviorally-based data collection and instructional system in place, and if they were to implement something different it would require training. Also Eddie's progress this year is off the charts with the behavioral and teaching methods currently in place. Mrs. Tracy has gone to the principal and is not backing down from wanting this method put in place—Soon! She has called for a new IEP and has ordered the videotapes of STAR and wants the staff to view them before the IEP.

How do you coach your staff on how to interact with Mrs. Tracy? How do you begin to shift Mrs. Tracy's perceptions about what constitutes appropriate teaching for her son to truly make her part of what appears to be a very solid classroom team?

Table 8–2. Frequency Data Form Example

Student	
Observer	
Date	
Target Behavior 1	Saying "hello" to peers
Target Behavior 2	Number of peers greeted
Target Behavior 3	

Time Period	Behavior 1	Behavior 2	Behavior 3
9:15–9:45	✓✓	✓	
9:45–10:15	✓	✓	
10:15–10:45			
10:45–11:15	✓	✓	
11:15–11:45			
11:45–12:15			
12:15–12:45	✓	✓	
12:45–1:15	✓✓✓	✓✓✓	
Total Incidents	8	7	

skills within an activity, simply counting the number of times the student engages in the activity will likely fail to provide an indication of which components of the activity have, and have not, been mastered. Last, when skills are intended to occur at a high frequency, it may be difficult for teachers and other adult staff to count every single instance of that behavior, thus leading to inaccuracies in the data collected. However, when a skill has a clear start and end and is performed within a relatively brief and consistent period of time, a frequency count can be an extremely efficient way to track student progress.

Interval Data Collection Methods

When the rate of a discrete skill (i.e., one with a clear start and end with relatively consistent duration) is high and thus difficult to track, utilizing an interval recording method can be useful. Interval data collection methods consist of determining a series of equal length intervals within which to track whether or not the targeted skill or behavior occurred. At the end of the data collection period, the percent of intervals in which the targeted skill or behavior occurred is calculated to provide a data point for that period. The formula used for this calculation is as follows:

$$\frac{\text{\# of intervals with an occurrence}}{\text{\# of total intervals}} \times 100 = \%$$

Thus, in the example provided in Table 8–3, the data point for Day 1 is 3/6 = 0.5, multiplied by 100 = 50%.

Duration Data Collection Methods

When the length of a targeted skill varies from one instance to the next, a duration recording method is typically appropriate. Duration recording simply involves recording the length of time that a skill, or skill set, is displayed. As such, a time-keeping device will need to be used by the data recorder, in addition to the data form itself. The length of each event of skill use is timed, and then placed on the form to be summed at the end of the recording period, thus generating the data point for that period. As seen in Table 8–4, duration allows for the analysis of student engagement in a targeted skill, or skill set, even when the length or rate of each event varies.

Latency Data Collection Methods

Another time-based data collection method is latency recording. Rather

Table 8–3. Interval Data Form Example

Student							
Observer							
Target Behavior	Initiation toward peers						
Interval (seconds):	0–30	31–60	61–90	91–120	121–150	151–180	%
Day 1	X	O	X	X	O	O	50%
Day 2	O	O	X	X	X	O	50%
Day 3	O	O	X	O	O	X	33%
Day 4	X	O	O	X	O	O	33%
Day 5	O	O	O	X	O	O	17%
Day 6							
Key	X = Occurrence (at least one occurrence within the interval) O = No occurrence						

Table 8–4. Duration Data Form Example

Student						
Observer						
Target Behavior	Sustaining Conversation With Peers					
Length of Time Behavior Occurred (in seconds)						
Date:	Event 1	Event 2	Event 3	Event 4	Event 5	Total:
Day 1	32	48	21	98	15	214 seconds
Day 2	24	15	57	NA	NA	96 seconds
Day 3	123	27	93	43	NA	286 seconds
Day 4	12	34	22	17	28	113 seconds
Day 5						

than recording the length of time a skill is performed, latency methods involve recording the length of time between a specific event (e.g., an instructional cue, a transition prompt, etc.) and an appropriate student response (e.g., a correct response, a successful transition, etc.). Latency recording can be helpful when the target of instruction is to increase response time, compliance with responding to adult direction, performing independent tasks, and so on. Similar to duration recording, a time-keeping device will need to be used in addition to the data form. Recording begins when the identified cue occurs, and ends when the student displays the criterion level of performance identified. So as indicated in Table 8–5, recording would begin when a peer greeted the student, and would end when the appropriate response was provided.

Task Analytic Data Collection Methods

When an area targeted for instruction consists of a multicomponent skill or a set of skills to be displayed within a multistep activity, particularly if a task analysis was conducted in order to determine the skills to be taught, a task analytic recording method should be utilized. Typically when multistep skill use is taught, adults will make use of evidence-based instruction involving various prompts and prompt fading methods. As such, task analytic recording methods need to account for different levels of prompts used for each step/skill to be displayed during the activity. As seen in Table 8–6, a key is used to illustrate which type of prompt was necessary for the student to display the step indicated successfully. As with

Table 8–5. Latency Data Form Example

Student						
Observer						
Target Behavior	Responding to a Greeting From a Peer					
Length of Time Until Behavior Occurred (in seconds)						
Date:	Event 1	Event 2	Event 3	Event 4	Event 5	Total:
Day 1	10	12	8	11	13	54 seconds
Day 2	10	8	5	6	5	34 seconds
Day 3	6	7	4	7	5	29 seconds
Day 4	4	4	5	3	2	18 seconds
Day 5	2	3	2	1	2	10 seconds

any prompt fading strategy, one would like to see the intensity of the prompts used decrease over time, indicating an increased level of independent performance of the skills. When generating a data point for each observation period, a criterion level of prompting will need to be determined prior to calculating the data point. Ideally, the criteria would be independent performance of the step/skill, as shown in Table 8–6, and calculated as the percentage of steps/skills performed independently (i.e., with no prompting necessary). However, for some students and/or in certain activities, prompts will need to be faded slowly, and it may take extended periods of time before independent performance will be observed. Yet if the data collection system is not sensitive to this (i.e., the criterion level is too high), one may miss gradual steady progress toward, albeit not yet reach-

ing, independent performance. For this reason, the criterion level can initially be set at various levels of prompts, such as "steps completed without physical prompting," whereby the percentage of steps/skills performed with any type of prompt other than a full or partial physical prompt would be calculated, as for example, the data displayed in Table 8–6.

Trials to Criterion Data Collection Methods

Evidence-based instructional strategies typically consist of numerous and ongoing instructional trials provided within activities over time. In order to monitor a student's progress in response to these instructional strategies, it is useful to record the student's level of accuracy when responding to instructional cues.

Table 8–6. Task Analytic Data Form Example

Student					
Observer					
Target Activity	Following a Visual Schedule				
Steps	Event 1	Event 2	Event 3	Event 4	Event 5
Step 1: Approach schedule	FP	FP	PP	PP	
Step 2: Remove top icon	FP	PP	PP	G	
Step 3: Take icon to indicated area/ activity	PP	PP	G	VP	
Step 4: Take icon to schedule (after activity)	FP	PP	VP	I	
Step 5: Place icon in pocket on schedule	VP	I	I	I	
Step 6: Select next icon	G	VP	I	I	
Daily Percent of Steps Completed Independently	0%	17%	33%	50%	
Key	FP = Full Physical Prompt PP = Partial Physical Prompt G = Gestural Prompt VP = Verbal Prompt I = Independent				

Hence, as displayed in Table 8–7, a "trials to criterion" data collection method can be employed whereby the student's response to each instructional trial is recorded during instruction. Again, as shown in Table 8–7, a key will need to be developed to indicate correct versus incorrect (and/or prompted) responses. It is important to note that most evidence-based instructional strategies involve much more than the five trials indicated on the form in Table 8–7. Instead, these data collection methods typically use a probe method, where data for only the first five trials of each instructional session are recorded. Last, with a "trials to criterion" method, a criterion level of satisfactory performance

Table 8–7. Trials to Criterion Data Form Example

Student					
Instructional Program	Pivotal Response Teaching				
Instructional Trials Addressed	Question-asking, "What's that?"				
Date/Session:	Session 1	Session 2	Session 3	Session 4	Session 5
Trial 1	I	I	C	C	C
Trial 2	I	C	I	C	C
Trial 3	C	C	C	C	C
Trial 4	C	I	C	C	C
Trial 5	I	C	C	C	C
Percentage	40%	60%	80%	100%	100%
Key	C = Correct Response I = Incorrect/Prompted Response				

must be established. This criterion level typically consists of both a performance level within a session, as well as a consecutive number of sessions in which the identified performance level must be displayed. So, for example, a criterion of 80% correct across three consecutive sessions, would be considered achieved or mastered performance in the sample form provided in Table 8–7.

Additional Considerations

A common question when collecting data is, "How much data should be collected?" As noted previously, data should only be collected when and if it directly informs instructional decision-making. When this is ensured, then the questions become more focused, such as, "Is the

instructional strategy working?"; "How long should instruction be delivered before decisions are made?"; or "When should we stop, change, or increase instruction?" In the upcoming sections the answers to these and other questions are addressed to provide a framework for coaches supporting teachers in their ongoing data collection, decision making, and instructional design, implementation, revision, and completion.

End-of-Chapter Questions

1. Complete the Team Checklist for Skill Selection Form (Table 8–1) for a student with ASD with whom you work. What skill received the highest ratings, and why? Could some of

the skill selection criteria be considered more important than others? Why, or why not?

2. Select one of the data collection forms provided in this chapter (see Tables 8–2 through 8–7) and practice collecting data on a behavior of your choice for a student with ASD.

3. Identify a multicomponent skill, and design a Task Analytic Data Collection Form to track the performance of that skill. Be sure to include each step in the task analysis, a prompt hierarchy and key for data entry, as well as a criterion level at which to calculate the percent of steps completed.

References

Brown, L., Nietupski, J., & Hamre Nietupski, S. (1976). The criterion of ultimate functioning and public school services for severely handicapped students. In M. A. Thomas (Ed.), *Hey, don't forget about me: New directions for serving the severely handicapped* (pp. 2–15). Reston, VA: Council for Exceptional Children.

Koegel, L. K., Koegel, R. L., Harrower, J. K., & Carter, C. M. (1999). Pivotal response intervention I: Overview of approach. *Journal of the Association for Persons with Severe Handicaps, 24*(3), 174–185.

National Standards Project. (2009). *Evidence-based practice and autism in the schools: A guide to providing appropriate interventions to students with autism spectrum disorders.* Randolph, MA: National Autism Center.

Schalock, R. L. (2004). The emerging disability paradigm and its implications for policy and practice. *Research and Practice for Persons with Severe Disabilities, 14,* 204–215.

Wehmeyer, M. L., Field, S., Doren, B., Jones, B., & Mason, C. (2004). Self-determination and student involvement in standards-based reform. *Exceptional Children, 70,* 413–425.

SECTION III

Using High-Quality Coaching to Deliver Effective Programming for Students With Autism Spectrum Disorder

Section III continues the discussion started in Section II about effective program and delves into the actual delivery of instruction utilizing evidence-based interventions (EBIs) to support students with autism spectrum disorder (ASD). Further details are provided on effective coaching supports for teachers when providing instruction in social communication skills, providing effective behavior supports and ensuring the development of skills and opportunities to ensure successful transition from school entry to exit, and beyond, to students with ASD. The last chapter describes how a school district can support a network of coaching leadership to better serve students with ASD. This culminating chapter elevates the notion of coaching to a level of importance so that a school district can provide incentives and resources to support this most important endeavor.

CHAPTER 9

Using High-Quality Coaching to Support the Delivery of Effective Instruction

I cannot emphasize enough the importance of a good teacher.
—Temple Grandin

Chapter Objectives

■ Present information for coaches and teachers on identifying evidence-based interventions (EBIs) for students with autism spectrum disorder (ASD).

■ Provide guidelines for coaches and teachers to follow when selecting instructional strategies for teaching meaningful skills to students with ASD.

■ Provide a model for coaches and teachers to use when collaborating to plan, deliver, and monitor evidence-based instruction.

Providing Evidence-Based Instruction

When selecting instructional strategies, it is imperative that the coach and the teacher are familiar with and select from strategies with an established evidence base demonstrating their effectiveness with students with ASD. Unfortunately, the history of the field of "autism interventions" is littered with high-profile fads, special diets, and other assorted cure-alls with, at best, no established effectiveness and, at worst, serious risk to the lives of children with ASD. More recent-ly, a number of instructional strategies have now been subjected to rigorous experimental evaluation and have demonstrated effectiveness in improving a broad range of meaningful skills leading to improved quality of life outcomes. Furthermore, these evidence-based interventions (EBIs) have been identified by a number of professional organizations that have made professional development resources for educators publicly available. Examples of these resources have been provided in Box 9–1, and the reader is encouraged to review these to enhance their familiarity with implementing specific EBIs.

Given the research findings and the widespread availability of professional development resources for educators on EBIs, it is no longer ethically defensible for educators to implement or advocate for unestablished treatments. Rather, coaches and teachers must make use of approaches that have a reasonable expectation of success. Yet, given the growing number of established instructional strategies, educators will need to make decisions about which EBIs to make use of when teaching particular skills. This may require a greater level of sophistication in order to match the instructional strategy to the skill area and instructional setting(s) in question.

Box 9–1. Professional Development Resources on Evidence-Based Interventions for Students With ASD

Autism Internet Modules from the Ohio Center for Autism and Low Incidence (OCALI):
http://www.autisminternetmodules.org

National Professional Development Center on Autism Spectrum Disorders:
http://autismpdc.fpg.unc.edu

National Autism Center's National Standards Project:
http://www.nationalautismcenter.org

UC, Davis MIND Institute's Education Resources:
http://www.ucdmc.ucdavis.edu/mindinstitute/resources/education.html

Given the range of skills that students with ASD may benefit from acquiring, and the variety of settings in which it would be desirable for these skills to be used, it is important to consider the full range of EBIs when selecting the strategy to implement. Furthermore, these strategies are not mutually exclusive and can, and often should, be combined in order to maximize outcomes.

Selecting the Instructional Setting(s)

After identifying the skill, or skills, to be taught, the next step in planning for the implementation of instruction is to deter-mine the setting, or settings, in which the identified skills will be taught. Considerations when selecting the instructional setting include the relevance and potential use of the skill in the setting, ecological factors or other external factors present in the setting that might affect the intervention, the availability of instructional materials and personnel in the setting, the capacity to incorporate student interest in the setting, the age appropriateness of the setting, and the expected duration of activities to occur in the setting. In order to determine the relative appropriateness of potential settings for instruction, the team can use a simple Instructional Setting Evaluation form, like the one in Table 9–1.

Table 9–1. Instructional Setting Evaluation Form

Name					
Date					
Target Skill(s)					
Scale	1 = No, 2 = Somewhat, 3 = Yes				
	Classroom	Playground	Cafeteria	Hallways	Other
Need for skill use	1 2 3	1 2 3	1 2 3	1 2 3	1 2 3
Freedom from distracting stimuli	1 2 3	1 2 3	1 2 3	1 2 3	1 2 3
Availability of materials/personnel	1 2 3	1 2 3	1 2 3	1 2 3	1 2 3
Ability to incorporate student interest	1 2 3	1 2 3	1 2 3	1 2 3	1 2 3
Age appropriateness	1 2 3	1 2 3	1 2 3	1 2 3	1 2 3
Adequacy for duration of instruction/activity	1 2 3	1 2 3	1 2 3	1 2 3	1 2 3
Total Score (out of 18)	/18	/18	/18	/18	/18

Determining the Intensity of Instruction

A number of considerations will need to be made by the team when determining "how much" instruction to provide. Certainly, the extent of a student's skill deficit will play a large role in this determination, because the greater the deficit, the more intensive the instruction will need to be. Therefore, it is important to map out the frequency (i.e., number of time per week) and duration (i.e., length of each instructional event) with which instruction in the targeted skill area will occur. However, additional considerations might include financial constraints, personnel availability, and availability of natural opportunities for instruction.

Arranging Opportunities for Instruction

Another important aspect of delivering effective instruction is to determine how to set up teaching opportunities. Three general categories of instructional "mode" can be considered. The first mode is individual direct instruc-tion, which typically consists of instruction delivered in a one-to-one adult to student format. A second mode is peer instruction, often characterized by an adult-facilitated interaction between the target student and a same-age, typically developing peer. The third mode, often referred to as milieu instruction, takes place during naturally occurring activities, typically involving multiple peers or group activities. These three instructional modes can probably be best viewed as a continuum, ranging from most to least adult directed. Thus, it may be helpful to plan for various combinations of instructional modes, taking advantage of the relative strengths of each. As Figure 9–1 indicates, individual modes of instruction have been associated with the acquisition of skills, and naturalistic modes of instruction have been associated with the generalization of those skills across settings, people, and instructional materials.

When involving peers in the instructional approach, a few considerations are in order. First, it may be helpful to prepare the peer, or peers, with both general information about disability or "ability awareness" (i.e., what is autism spectrum disorder?), as well as the specific strengths and needs of the student

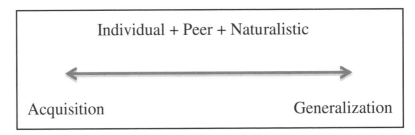

Figure 9–1. Modes of instruction.

with ASD (e.g., "Carlos loves trains, but sometimes has trouble inviting friends to play with him."). Second, the specific role as peer partner in instruction will be helpful (e.g., "I'd like you to help Carlos learn how to ask friends to play. To do this, I will ask you to . . . "). Last, considerations for motivating peers to participate should be made, such as selecting highly preferred activities, as well as a reward system for participation.

Regardless of the mode(s) selected for instruction, it will be critical to determine which adult(s) will provide, or facilitate, the instruction (e.g., teacher, aide, speech-language pathologist [SLP], etc.). In order to maximize generalization, multiple instructors and/or social partners will be necessary. One may choose to start with a single instructor delivering individual instruction to ensure skill acquisition, and then systematically introduce new instructors and partners, particularly when incorporating more naturalistic modes of instruction to promote generalization.

Ensuring Motivation

Last, while motivational strategies are built into most EBIs, it is important to consider strategies for enhancing student motivation to participate in instruction on an ongoing basis. Strategies such as incorporating student choice, utilizing highly preferred activities, varying tasks, interspersing previously mastered instructional trials, and implementing differential reinforcement strategies throughout instruction will maximize student engagement in instruction.

Monitoring Progress

Selecting from among established EBIs enhances the likelihood that student outcomes will be achieved, but a common element to utilizing EBIs is to actively monitor the student's progress in response to the instructional method. Knowing how the student is responding to the instruction being provided will allow educators to decide when instructional outcomes have been achieved, or when to change instructional approaches due to lack of progress. A common data collection strategy used to maximize efficient progress monitoring is the use of data probes. Data probes consist of collecting consistent but intermittent data during instruction. So, for example, an instructor implementing a Discrete Trial Teaching approach may collect data on just the first five trials of each instructional session, rather than for every trial. As a result, data probes provide a reliable estimate of overall student progress while simultaneously allowing instructors to deliver instruction without the continuous interruption of filling out data forms. Given that the primary reason for collecting data is to make valid instructional decisions, the data collected will need to be presented in a way to enhance the ability of the team to do this. This typically involves the creation of line graphs, allowing for quick visual inspection of student progress. As seen in Figure 9–2, the features of a line graph include a title describing what the graph is intended to show; a *y*-axis indicating the data collection method used and a label for the skill

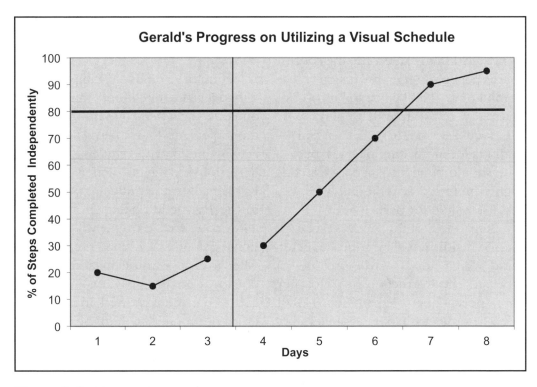

Figure 9–2. Line graph example.

being tracked; an *x*-axis indicating the time frame over which data was collected; and finally, data points plotted on the graph and connected by lines to represent the student's progress.

Additionally, a vertical phase line can be inserted to indicate baseline versus instructional phases. Another key feature of the graph presented in Figure 9–2 is the horizontal goal line, placed at the 80% level. Including a goal line on the graph itself enhances the ease with which to quickly determine when instructional outcomes have been met. Note that additional phases can be added to the graph as the student begins to progress in generalizing acquired skills to new situations.

Consultative Coaching (CC) Example on Providing Instruction

The "Fitting In" vignette in Box 9–2 provides a scenario where consultative coaching would be extremely helpful in designing a set of effective instructional strategies.

Because Ngyuen's problem occurred in unstructured social situations with peers, the coach and school SLP agreed that the social rules about greeting strangers needed to be embedded in an activity that would re-create the dynamics of greeting someone who was unfamiliar. Video self-modeling was selected,

---

Box 9–2. Vignette: Fitting In

Ngyuen was a teenager with ASD and strong adaptive skills. He arrived from another country at the age of 14 and was completing his freshman year in high school in the United States. Ngyuen's challenges in social communication were brought to the attention of an HQC-A. The school psychologist described Ngyuen as lacking an ability to understand and respond to important cues from his peers, failing to adjust his behavior to their reaction to his social overtures. The speech-language pathologist who supported Ngyuen in a small social skills group, had worked on explicit social rules when greeting others and rules for where to stand in proximity to another person. But this skill was not generalizing when Ngyuen attended his mainstream classes; often he would approach unfamiliar students with gestures that were physically intrusive and silly. His parents noted that much of his behavioral difficulties stemmed from his intense desire to fit in at school and to have friendships; however, they lamented that ultimately peers "don't like him" and would flee from him.

　The coach observed Ngyuen in less-structured school activities like physical education, as this was where many of his social challenges occurred. She observed that as the teacher's verbal instructions about an upcoming activity lengthened, Ngyuen's anxiety increased; he was quickly out of his seat pacing back and forth, and using a great deal of self-talk. Ngyuen was able to regroup as students transitioned to the track and field area; however, he suddenly approached an unfamiliar male student and draped his arm over the student's shoulder, greeting him with "How's it going?" Even though the student tried several times to extricate himself, Ngyuen appeared unaware of the many nonverbal signals from the student that this behavior was making him uncomfortable.

---

as this evidence-based practice has been used successfully with ASD students in modifying social behavior (Maione & Mirenda, 2006; Nikopoulos & Nikopoulou-Smyrni, 2008). The SLP previewed an activity for the group where students reenacted the "right way" and the "wrong way" to greet someone whom they did not know well on campus. One student operated a hand-held digital camera, while the others role-played a greeting using body language signals that unambiguously communicated their dislike if the other partner violated their personal space or the expected rules of interaction; for example, if a partner tried to grab someone by the forearm. When Ngyuen practiced the first time, he forgot the social rule and walked up to and hugged the SLP. To address this additional challenge, another evidence-based strategy, social narratives, was implemented to augment the video modeling exercise. The resulting narrative, "Meeting People I Don't Know Well" was formatted in a presentation mode on a computer and illustrated with graphics depicting the expected social rules.

As the narrative in Box 9–3 clarifies, the rule about standing a comfortable distance away from an unfamiliar conversational partner, referred to as "personal distance area," was at the crux of Ngyuen's perspective-taking challenges. He inaccurately perceived that all peers were social partners willing to be greeted effusively. To additionally reinforce the personal distance area rule, the SLP and coach found a graphic image that explained the rule with a detailed illustration: "My personal area; don't stand in it." The illustration portrayed a comic stick figure standing with outstretched arms within a cylinder bounded by a three-to-five-feet area with the text: "I belong here." Outside of that boundary, additional text read: "You belong here."

This graphic made explicit what a reasonable personal distance area was depending on the degree of the social partners' familiarity with one another. Ngyuen was successful in reenacting the rule in a follow-up video self-modeling

---

Box 9–3. Meeting People I Don't Know Well

At high school many people don't know one another very well. Usually, when they pass in the halls, they don't greet one another. Sometimes, when people who don't know one another pass in the halls, they may extend their hand and say "hello?" People who don't know one another will keep their personal distance area (PDA) about 8 to 12 feet apart when they greet each other. If they are close friends their PDA might be closer than 8 to 12 feet. Usually, they stand 2 to 3 feet apart and might clasp hands, or bump fists to say "hello." People who don't know one another very well remember to practice their PDA; that way they feel comfortable. I will try to remember the PDA at school, too, so people who don't know me well will feel comfortable about me.

session. His therapist replayed the video to help him generalize what he was able to perform in this structured scenario. Eventually he was able to generalize this skill in his mainstream classes and school extracurricular activities.

End-of-Chapter Questions

1. Special education teachers working with students with ASD are often asked by others (family members, advocates, related service providers) to implement strategies that are not evidence based. Imagine that you have been asked by a parent of one of your students to implement a strategy that is not evidence based for students with ASD. How would you respond to such a request?

2. Complete the Instructional Setting Evaluation Form (see Table 9–1) for a student you work with. Which setting received the highest ratings, and why? Could some of the setting evaluation criteria be considered

more important than others? Why, or why not?

3. Create an example of a line graph displaying progress for a hypothetical student with ASD. Determine a skill to be targeted, the data collection method used, and plot hypothetical data on the graph. Be sure to include all of the relevant features of a line graph, as described in this chapter and as seen in Figure 9–2.

References

Maione, L., & Mirenda, P. (2006). Effects of video modeling and video feedback on peer-directed social language skills of a child with autism. *Journal of Positive Behavior Interventions, 8*(2), 106–118.

Nikopoulos, C., & Nikopoulou-Smyrni, P. (2008). Teaching complex social skills to children with autism: Advances of video modeling. *Journal of Early and Intensive Behavior Intervention, 5*(2), 30–43.

Westling, D. L., & Fox, L. L. (2009). *Teaching students with severe disabilities* (4th ed.). New York, NY: Pearson Education.

CHAPTER 10

Coaching the Instruction of Social Communication Skills

*The difference between the right word and the almost right word
is the difference between lightning and a lightning bug.*
                                                    —Mark Twain

---

Chapter Objectives

■ Review the justification to prioritize social communication instruction for students with autism spectrum disorder (ASD).

■ Highlight some of the research examining the effectiveness of teaching social communication skills to individuals with ASD.

■ Describe several evidence-based interventions (EBIs) for supporting social communication at different skill levels.

■ Provide case examples and ways in which high-quality coaches can support teachers in the implementation of EBIs for social communication.

Introduction

Throughout this book, we have justified why high-quality coaching is ideal for supporting teaching teams and service providers who instruct students with ASD. Whether novice or more veteran in their experience, teachers benefit from coaching opportunities to learn about the complexities of this disorder and how to comprehensively provide a range of high-quality instruction. Compared to one-time professional development trainings, expert coaching is an optimal way to establish and sustain evidence-based instruction for teachers and therapists working with students whose needs are multidimensional and complex. In this chapter, we extend discussion about one of the primary core deficits challenging individuals on the spectrum, social communication, and ways in which coaches can effectively scaffold it for instructional teams. An overarching theme in this chapter aligns with best-practice guidelines for educating young children with ASD (National Autism Center, 2015; Wong et al., 2014) (see Chapter 2). One principal guideline is that family values as well as priorities of the educational team are balanced. For example, having a child learn to request his or her preferred meal at a restaurant or a favorite television show is equally as important as working on specific communication skills in the classroom setting. Best-practice guidelines emphasize that instruction should focus on spontaneous communication in functional activities within different learning environments (home, school, community) and ensure that the individual with ASD interacts with different communicative partners, including typically developing age peers, to achieve skill generalization.

The organization of this chapter is structured to include strategies that align with a continuum of evidence-based interventions (EBIs) identified by the National Professional Development Center (NPDC) for Autism Spectrum Disorders (Wong et al., 2014) and the National Standards Project (NSP) for ASD (National Autism Center, 2015). The reader is encouraged to investigate these reports to acquire a comprehensive knowledge base about the criteria for inclusion of treatment studies in the NPDC and NSP reports regarding how EBIs compare and contrast and how they should be systematically implemented. Consistent with the common core deficits of ASD identified in Section I (see Chapter 2), we emphasize interventions that address the core area of social communication.

Why Focus on Social Communication?

Why is it so vital to focus on social communication for individuals with ASD? Understanding this core deficit is paramount for coaches and teachers if they are to assist students in building social relationships to ultimately help them succeed as adults. Because social communication so pervasively impacts human relationships across the life span for individuals with ASD, it requires intensive and systematic intervention from an early age well into adolescence and young adulthood. As detailed in Chapter 2, the *DSM-5* identifies three symptom areas encompassing this core challenge: (a) developing, maintaining, and understanding relationships; (b) establishing social-emotional reciprocity; and (c) using nonverbal communicative behaviors for social interaction (APA, 2013). Broad categories on which to focus the implementation of evidence-based practices can be broken down as follows: (a) teaching initial communication and expanding upon existing communication skills (e.g., initiating, responding, elaborating, etc.) and (b) improving the social, or pragmatic, use of language (e.g., play, peer interactions, social skills, etc.). Furthermore, EBIs can be characterized in two different ways: comprehensive intervention programs and specific intervention strategies. The following sections will provide information on, and examples of these two types of EBIs which have been found to be so critical in improving social communication skills for students with ASD.

Coaching Teachers to Provide Comprehensive Evidence-Based Instruction in Addressing Social Communication Skills for Students With ASD

A long history of research, particularly in the field of applied behavior analysis (ABA), has resulted in the identification of effective comprehensive strategies for improving the communication skills of students with ASD (NAC, 2015). *Comprehensive* EBIs are characterized by a wide-ranging applicability to address the full range of social communication (and behavioral) needs of students with ASD. Two comprehensive intervention approaches, currently considered best practice for teaching a host of initial communication skills as well as for expanding the complexity of existing communication skills for students with ASD (Wong et al., 2014) are Discrete Trial Teaching (DTT) (Smith, 2001) and Pivotal Response Treatment (PRT) (Koegel & Koegel, 2012).

Discrete Trial Teaching: Implications for Coaches and Teachers of Students With ASD

Discrete Trial Teaching (DTT) methods are characterized by individualized and simplified forms of instruction, consisting of distinct instructional events, or trials, delivered in rapid succession (Smith, 2001). Thus, students with ASD are provided with many opportunities (e.g., trials) to practice specific communication skills and receive feedback from the instructor. Each instructional trial consists of critical components known to improve learning, even among students severely impacted by ASD. These components are to be provided by the instructor in the sequence shown in Figure 10–1.

As can be seen in Figure 10–1, DTT begins with capturing the student's attention in order to ensure that the student is attending to the instructional event. Capturing the student's attention

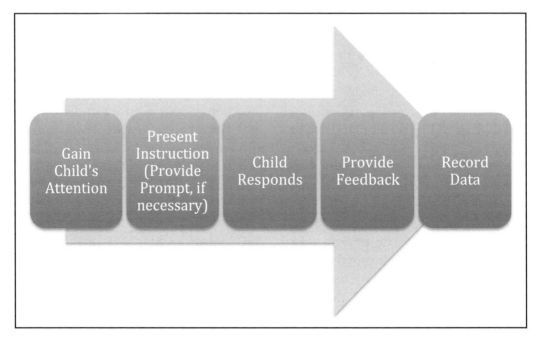

Figure 10–1. Components of an instructional trial used in discrete trial teaching.

can be achieved by delivering a verbal cue (e.g., saying the child's name, saying "Look," etc.), a gestural cue (e.g., the instructor pointing to the materials), or simply waiting for the student to make eye contact. Once the student is attending, the instructional cue is delivered (e.g., showing a picture card and asking, "What's this?"). Instructional cues should be brief, direct, and delivered only once before the next component of instruction occurs. If the instructional trial is focused on teaching an initial skill, it may be necessary for the instructor to provide an additional prompt to increase the likelihood that the student will respond correctly. This prompt might immediately follow the instructional cue (e.g., Instructional Cue: "What's this?" Prompt: "Ball!"). Following delivery of the instructional cue, and the prompt if necessary, the next component involves providing an opportunity for the student to respond (e.g, student says, "Ball"). Typically a time delay procedure is used here, whereby the instructor waits for a specified period of time (e.g., 3 to 5 seconds) to allow the student to respond. Then the next step is to deliver feedback based upon the student's response. If for example, the student's response was correct (e.g., the picture card did display a ball), then reinforcement is immediately delivered. Reinforcement should always include behavior-specific praise (e.g., "Yes it's a ball, nice talking!"), but may also be paired with something determined to be more motivating for the student (e.g., small edibles, a high five, etc.), or even via the use of a token board, as described in the next chapter (see Chapter 11). If the student does not respond within the time frame, or gives an incorrect response, then the instructor refrains from saying anything in response, and instead clears the field of any instructional materials, waits a few seconds, and reintroduces the original instructional cue again. Sometimes it is helpful to follow this error correction strategy by immediately delivering a few quick instructional trials in a skill previously mastered by the student (e.g., "Touch your nose," "Give me five," etc.), or a maintenance trial, just prior to reintroducing the instructional trial that the student did not respond to correctly. The last component of DTT is to record data on the student response (see Chapter 8, Table 8–7 for a sample recording form). Typically this would involve the instructor indicating if the student response was (a) correct, (b) correct with an additional prompt provided, or (c) incorrect. Given the high number of instructional trials that may be delivered in a DTT session, collecting data on the first few trials of each session, as a probe, can serve as an efficient way to get an estimate of student progress.

Although recommendations regarding the amount of DTT to be provided vary, in order for the student with ASD to acquire initial, and certainly expanded, expressive and receptive communication skills, a high number of hours per week are typically required (Smith, 2001). Furthermore, a high level of training is required in order for teachers and support personnel to become proficient in implementing DTT approaches. Thus, a teacher learning to implement DTT would likely require intensive coaching (IC) to set up effective programming in

this area. Given the intensive level of support that many students with ASD will need in order to develop initial and expanded communication skills, investing in the training and coaching of both coaches and teachers to implement DTT approaches is often made a priority by district offices of special education.

Pivotal Response Treatment: Implications for Coaches and Teachers of Students With ASD

Like DTT, Pivotal Response Treatment (PRT) makes use of the individualized and simplified instructional strategies derived from the field of ABA. However, PRT is typically characterized by its focus on improving social communicative outcomes in key skill areas known to also result in improvements in untargeted skills (Koegel, Koegel, Harrower, & Carter, 1999). These *pivotal skills* are also often targeted for improvement in typical natural settings, activities, and routines in which the skills would ultimately need to be used independently by the student with ASD (e.g., classrooms, playground, meals, etc.). Learning variables that have been demonstrated to be effectively targeted via PRT approaches include student motivation, responding to multiple cues, self-management, and self-initiations (Koegel & Koegel, 2012). Although a detailed discussion on each of these pivotal areas is beyond the scope of this chapter (readers are referred to Koegel & Koegel, 2006, 2012 for thorough descriptions of the PRT approach), we briefly outline the pivotal area of student motivation as it relates to coaches and teachers working to support the social communication of students with ASD.

In the context of PRT, student motivation has been characterized by increases in attempts to respond to instruction, decreased delay in responding (i.e., response latency), and improved emotional affect (eye contact, smiles, orientation toward instructor and materials) (Koegel et al., 1999). Thus, when strategies focused on increasing motivation during instruction are implemented, student acquisition and generalization of skills improves as well (Koegel, O'Dell, & Koegel, 1987). When targeting the pivotal area of motivation, it is important to incorporate the following strategies: (a) child choice, (b) natural and direct reinforcers, (c) interspersing maintenance trials, and (d) reinforcing attempts. When it comes to incorporating child choice during instruction, one of the ways in which this is implemented is by following the student's lead in the selection of instructional materials. So if a teacher who is working on providing instruction to a student on making verbal requests observes the student walking over to a container of toys, the teacher could provide an instructional cue for the student to request assistance in opening the container, using the same time delay procedures and prompts, if necessary, as used in DTT (e.g., "What do you want to play with?"). The teacher could then also provide instructional cues prompting the student to request the toy the student is interested in (e.g., "Car"). Subsequent instructional trials can then be delivered around the use of the toy in a play activity (e.g., turn-taking, pretend play, etc.). The second strategy involves the use of natural and direct reinforcers. In the above example, getting access to the toy itself, which is contingent on the student requesting it, exemplifies a natural and direct reinforcer as there is a natural relationship between the behavior and the reinforcing item (i.e., requesting "car" results in access to the toy car). Next, the use of instructional trials previously mastered by the student throughout instructional sessions can maintain student motivation allowing for an increase in length of engagement in instructional activities. Thus, for example, during the instruction focused on teaching the requesting of a student-selected item (e.g. toy car), the teacher could intersperse instructional trials focused on previously acquired receptive communication skills (e.g., "lift the car up"). Last, rather than making reinforcement contingent on a perfectly correct response, strategies incorporating student motivation provide reinforcement following reasonable attempts to respond (e.g., if the student requests the toy car by saying the initial sound /k/ in the word "car," the teacher provides access to the car). Over time these responses are shaped to more fully exemplify appropriate responses, by gradually increasing the criteria for reinforcement. So in the example provided in this section, after mastering the initial /k/ sound in "car," the instructor would then make access to the toy car contingent on the student saying /ka/, and ultimately make it contingent on saying the full word "car."

In addition to documented improvements in the initial development of communication, and the expansion of existing communication skills, PRT has been demonstrated to be effective in addressing difficulties around the pragmatic or social use of language among students with ASD (Koegel & Frea, 1993; Koegel, Park, & Koegel, 2014; Pierce & Schreibman, 1997), even when teaching complex social communicative skills (Pierce & Schreibman, 1995). As with the DTT approach, teachers may require intensive coaching (IC) supports to fully implement a comprehensive PRT approach. However, as noted in the example above for student motivation (and as described in Chapter 11 with regard to Self-Management), a number of key strategies derived from the research on PRT can also be incorporated into daily instruction with support provided via peer-to-peer (PtP) or consultative coaching (CC).

Coaching Teachers to Provide Specific Evidence-Based Strategies in Addressing Social Communication Skills for Students With ASD

A number of specific intervention strategies have been demonstrated to be effective in addressing the social communication needs of students with ASD (NAC, 2015; Wong et al., 2014). These strategies are characterized as *specific* due to the fact that they will often be implemented along with other specific or comprehensive strategies to support the full range of social communication needs that a student with ASD would be likely to display. The following sections provide information and examples for coaches and teachers on a sampling of these specific evidence-based interventions.

Coaching the Instruction of Social Communication Skills Using Peer-Mediated Interventions

An established intervention for supporting social communication is peer-mediated instruction (PMI). With this EBI, typically developing peers are taught explicit strategies to facilitate play and social interaction with targeted students with ASD. Ideally, PMI is frequently carried out in inclusive settings, where there are ample opportunities to model, prompt, and practice skills in natural social contexts (e.g., recess, lunch, hallways, assemblies, club meetings). Peers have been successfully taught by SLPs, school psychologists, and teachers to initiate and maintain topics, establish greetings, answer questions, comment on joint activities, and use other self-monitoring strategies with targeted students (Thiemann-Bourque, 2010). Integrated Play Groups is a peer-training intervention approach in which small groups of typically developing children, including children with ASD and their siblings, play under the guidance of an adult facilitator (Wolfberg & Schuler, 1993). The goal is to increase the target child's motivation to regularly socialize with typically developing peers.

Studies examining PMI have reported favorable outcomes for improving a variety of social skills in students with ASD, increasing their variety and rate of communicative initiations and responsiveness (Chan et al., 2009), as well as improved teacher ratings of students' pro-social skills (Kamps et al., 2015). However, there are challenges, such as ensuring that peer partners are consistent in their standard application of strategies and dosage of use. Research has questioned whether PMI is adequate on its own to improve social competence in ASD, or whether additional supportive strategies make a critical difference in the acquisition and maintenance of specific social communication skills. A few studies have found that enhancing PMIs with written text cues (written phrases of what to say), picture cues of students engaging in social interaction, and sociodramatic scripts significantly enhances these outcomes for individuals with ASD (Goldstein, Schneider, & Thiemann, 2007; Thiemann & Goldstein, 2004). These investigators found that visual and text supports provided subjects with access to a means of understanding a dynamically changing set of social cues, including facial expression, gesture, tone of voice, and physical proximity of a partner.

Coaching the Instruction of Social Communication Skills Using Video Modeling

Video modeling (VM) consists of presenting a video recording to the student with ASD in which a model engaging in a target behavior is depicted, with the opportunity for subsequent imitation of the model by the student (Maione & Mirenda, 2006). Video modeling offers a way to learn through social models without initial face-to-face interactions, which can be preferable for many students with autism (Corbett & Abdullah, 2005). Selective attention in response to VM is thought to improve because of repeated exposure to static and dynamic visual cues that individuals with ASD can focus on (Corbett & Abdullah, 2005). In addition, retention is increased with opportunities for practice and repeated viewing of the video media.

A meta-analysis of VM research concluded that VM is an effective intervention strategy for improving social communication skills, functional skills, and behavioral functioning in children with ASD, and meet criteria for consideration as an evidence-based practice (Bellini & Akullian, 2007). Research has demonstrated the effectiveness of VM procedures in teaching a variety of different skills in the area of social communication, including conversational speech (Charlop & Milstein, 1989), communication (Baharov & Darling, 2007), peer-directed social language skills (Maione & Mirenda, 2006), social initiation and complex social interactions (Nikopolous & Nicopoulou-Smyrni, 2008), and generalization of skills in play activities (Paterson & Arco, 2007). Many of these studies have investigated video modeling's effectiveness with a wide range of students across many different age groups (Bellini & Akullian, 2007).

Combining Specific EBIs for Social Communication: An Example of Video Modeling and Peer-Mediated Instruction

As mentioned previously, specific EBIs can be combined in order to maximize their effectiveness and appropriateness to the needs of the student with ASD. A successful implementation of combining of the two specific EBIs just discussed (VM and PMI) appears in the vignette about Miguel (Box 10–1) and in the description that follows.

The school district hired a high-quality coach–autism (HQC-A) to coach the school SLP working with Miguel as well as his Individualized Education Program (IEP) team. The HQC-A's first objective was to observe Miguel in class and on the playground, and meet with the family to share observations and identify their major concerns and goals for their son. Following the family interview, the coach met with the SLP to brainstorm new IEP goals that reflected family priorities for peer socialization. Although Miguel's existing speech-language goals focused on improving his production of the /s/ sound, social communication goals were added:

1. Miguel will establish friendships with peers, who share interests as

---

Box 10–1. Vignette: Miguel

Miguel is a student with high-functioning autism fully included in Mrs. Pinneli's second-grade classroom. He is achieving at grade level in all academic subjects and does well with peers except for his awkward social communication with them. Miguel's fluent vocabulary and grammar are overall language strengths; however, he has difficulty changing topics in conversations with peers and accurately understanding their perspective. According to his teacher, when there is a breakdown in communication, he often gives up explaining things, walks away, or retreats to his desk and pulls out a workbook to look at.

Miguel has few playmates his own age at school. Instead, he prefers to join kindergarten students at recess. If left on his own, Miguel plays on playground equipment avoiding any interaction whatsoever with his classmates. His parents are understandably concerned that unless this pattern changes, Miguel will have a difficult time succeeding in upper elementary grades, where social demands and friendships become more complex.

evidenced by repeated social interaction with peers in structured group activities.

2. Miguel will persist and repair communicative breakdowns by modifying his language and behavior in four out of five conversational opportunities in the classroom.

To implement the first goal, the SLP and coach selected two specific EBIs: peer-mediated training and video modeling. In the first stage of peer-mediated training, three familiar peers, who were strong social models, were recruited to join a recess playgroup. Peers were individually coached that "they were needed to help Miguel make friends at recess." Then they practiced modeling and prompting of greetings, turn-taking, and topic continuation strategies (making comments, asking questions, and giving compliments) with the SLP and coach. The SLP and coach instructed Miguel and his peer group, asking them to come up with a list of steps and a script for playing a game at recess; they produced the following: (a) find a friend(s) to play with; (b) say "hello" and say your name: "Hi, I'm Miguel"; (c) invite your friend(s) to play: "Do you want to play with me?"; (d) decide on what to play: "Let's play dodge ball"; (e) decide on the rules of the game; (f) play the game; and (g) end the game: "Goodbye, see you at the next recess" (Figure 10–2).

In the second phase of implementation, video modeling, the group took turns rehearsing the script while it was video-recorded by the SLP. The coach edited the video adding text to clarify the seven steps, and the next

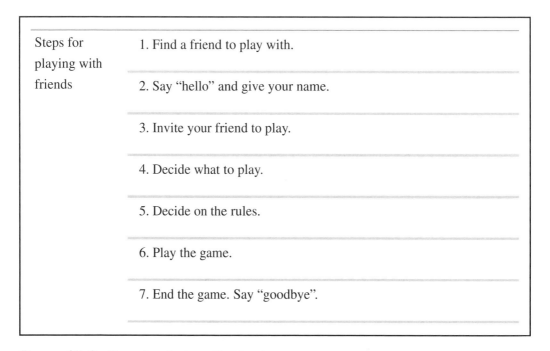

Steps for playing with friends	1. Find a friend to play with.
	2. Say "hello" and give your name.
	3. Invite your friend to play.
	4. Decide what to play.
	5. Decide on the rules.
	6. Play the game.
	7. End the game. Say "goodbye".

Figure 10–2. Steps for playing with friends.

day replayed the video for Miguel and peers. Both SLP and coach joined them on the playground and video-recorded the recess group as they enacted the seven steps. To ensure maintenance of this play skill, an instructional assistant observed Miguel daily and logged his social interactions with peers at recess. She kept a frequency count of the number of incidences of targeted social skills listed in Table 10–1. As data indicate, asking a friend to play, initiating a conversation, and other social interactions increased over the 5-day period. Miguel's frequency of joining an ongoing game declined from the first few days, but this was because he was inviting his friend(s) to play a new game and initiating conversation about the game rules. Data from Table 10–1 showed that when play ended, Miguel did not communicate leave-taking with "goodbye" or some other appropriate communicative signal. The SLP and HQC-A felt that this skill could be modeled and prompted by peers when opportunities arose, and

thus, that became the next target of his social communication intervention.

One of the successful ways in which the SLP changed her service delivery for Miguel was to provide support in his general education classroom during instructional time. The advantage was seeing how and to what extent Miguel engaged with peers in the classroom. The SLP was then able to effectively address the second goal relating to repairing communicative breakdowns in naturally occurring activities with peers. Initially, one peer was invited into a dyad with Miguel, where they practiced the "Barrier Game." Miguel and peer were given identical sets of materials (e.g., pieces of paper clothing to dress five drawings of snowmen). A physical barrier (trifold file) was placed on a small table, so that each partner could not see what the other was doing. Using materials on his side of the barrier, Miguel arranged the materials and verbally described how the snowmen should be dressed so that his partner could match his descriptions

Table 10–1. Frequency of Social Interactions at Recess Over Consecutive Days for Miguel

Days	Joined Ongoing Game	Invited Friend to Play	Started Conversation	Ended Conversation	Social Interaction Observed
1		xx	xx		x
2		x	x		x
3		xx	xx	x	x
4	x	x	x	x	x
5	x				x

Note. x = an occurrence of the targeted skill.

(e.g., "The first snowman has a purple scarf and a dotted hat"). When there were mismatches, Miguel was asked to repair this communicative breakdown using the critical missing element (e.g., "The last snowman has a *red* scarf"). The SLP and coach videotaped this activity and replayed it for Miguel and his partner. Eventually, communicative repair strategies were embedded into new activities (e.g., asking someone to repeat a message that was too soft, or was distorted and misunderstood with Miguel and his peers), which encouraged Miguel to employ comprehension monitoring and communicative repair strategies (see Dollaghan & Kaston, 1986; Merrison & Merrison, 2005).

Coaching the Instruction of the Social Use of Language Using Social Scripts and Narratives

Embedding social scripts into daily activities and routines for students with ASD has been demonstrated to be effective in increasing social use of language with peers (Sarokoff, Taylor, & Poulson, 2001). Social scripts are textual, pictorial, or audio prompts focusing on specific communication targets (e.g., initiations, greetings, conversational phrases, etc.), which students are taught to use during an activity involving a communicative partner, typically a peer (Garcia-Albea, Reeve, Brothers, & Reeve, 2014). Once students learn to use the communication target(s) outlined in the social script, its use is gradually faded to the point where the student is able to perform the skill without prompting or further use

of the script. The use of social scripts has not only resulted in the independent use of the communication skills targeted directly by the script, but has also generalized to unscripted, spontaneous communication in untargeted social activities and routines (Krantz & McClannahan, 1998).

Similar to social scripts, social narratives provide support to students with autism in using social communication skills with others during typical activities and routines. Social narratives, however, are characterized by longer textual passages, often with information provided that is intended to enhance a student's understanding of a communicative partner's potential perspective during a targeted activity (Collet-Klingenberg & Franzone, 2008). One promising social narrative approach for teaching social communication to students with ASD is an intervention originally proposed by Gray and Garand (1993) and published as Social Stories™. Social Stories, like other social narratives, teach social referencing (perspective taking) as well as a host of other social communication skills. A social narrative is a short script designed in a specific format that describes a situation, perspective, or expectation that is challenging for the student to understand or follow. The aim of the story is to share accurate information in an easily understood format and to offer opportunities for individuals to rehearse the narrative with adult support. Adolescents and young adults with advanced language skills seem particularly able to benefit from this support.

Despite questions about the effectiveness of social narratives in less controlled settings like the home, and what

---

Box 10–2. Vignette: Sarah

Sarah had recently been diagnosed with high-functioning ASD in her freshman year at a public high school. She had above-average language and intellectual skills for her age, but her social interpersonal skills were exceptionally delayed. Sarah's problem was that she would have unexpected meltdowns in her classes. She did not participate successfully with peers in cooperative group activities and seemed clueless about a number of expectations for participating appropriately in class. Sarah's parents explained that at an early age, preschool teachers noticed her social withdrawal and challenging behaviors that ultimately resulted in ejection from three private preschools and private school in the first grade. Because of her difficult behavioral issues, Sarah was home-schooled by her grandmother, and over years of instruction acquired academic skills that were at or above grade level. She was an avid reader and loved the sciences, so when her parents moved to another city, they decided to try enrolling her in public school again where her social problems were striking. Having never learned how to raise her hand to be recognized, Sarah impulsively blurted out answers to questions in class, often walking to the front of the room to interrupt a teacher during lecture. In her physics laboratory class, Sarah threw a tantrum when experiments did not go as planned and collapsed under the lab table curled up in a ball on the floor. Her physics teacher demanded that for safety's sake, she get up off the floor, yet the more he insisted on appropriate social behavior, the more Sarah regressed. On most days, she coped by taking out a novel to read during class time refusing to participate further. Desperate for ways to know how to instruct Sarah, her IEP case manager and general education teachers asked the director of Special Programs for support. The situation was so compelling, an HQC-A was asked to observe and meet with the instructional team as soon as possible.

---

frequency of exposure (dose) is optimal for skill maintenance, a number of studies have shown significant and positive outcomes for students introduced to this intervention (Karkhaneh et al., 2010; Wong et al., 2014). Social narratives provide the individual with opportunity to rehearse a prewritten script in a controlled setting with explicit identification of the context cues important for successful social interaction. A narrative may call attention to the physical environment and/or social partners present (e.g., "At school, recess, church; with my teacher, Mom, Dad"), explain social norms such as waiting for a clerk to take an order, sitting quietly in a doctor's office, suggest problem-solving alternatives (e.g., "I can sit somewhere else"), or mention another individual's perspectives (e.g., "He may be thinking that I'm a stranger.") (Gray, 2010). A social narrative may also identify the component steps for successfully undertaking an activity that is not well established in the student's repertoire, such as practicing a recently taught skill (e.g., terminating a conversation or introducing a change in topic).

Having never been to public school where the rules of social participation are inculcated at an early age, Sarah, a high school student recently identified with autism spectrum disorder, was challenged by a lack of exposure to cooperative learning experiences with peers (see vignette in Box 10–2). Following extended observation in her physics class and interviews with the IEP team, an HQC-A suggested to the team that support strategies capitalize on Sarah's strong desire to participate in science education and to read. The coach provided the teaching staff with a brief training on evidence-based social skill interventions for ASD. She asked team members to problem solve a support strategy addressing Sarah's behavior in physics lab. The team collectively drafted a social narrative (Box 10–3) to

---

Box 10–3. Sample Social Story: Group Work in Physics Lab

I go to physics lab on Thursday afternoons. Usually, I work in groups in my physics lab. The goal of working in this group is to understand the principles of physics, and take turns sharing what we have learned with one another in the group. We usually complete an experiment together and report on the results in class, or in our lab journals.

Sometimes, experiments don't work the way they were expected to. Experiments can fail, or the principles we're learning about don't fit with the results. When this happens, I usually feel frustrated. I can try to stay calm (by breathing in and out) and stay seated in my chair when this happens. When experiments don't go as expected, I can remember that this is how scientists have corrected their theories.

It is a good idea to stay calm in physics lab, because I will be able to learn better and think more clearly about principles and respond to my teacher and friends in class.

highlight the expectations of working in a group. Additionally, the narrative was illustrated with relevant visual supports (e.g., photographs of Einstein and a group of high school teens working collaboratively).

Sarah was introduced to this narrative before she went to lab and was able to clarify her understanding of the script's content or other unexpected issues with the case manager. Thereafter, she reviewed it weekly. Her physics teacher graphically recorded any incidences of Sarah falling to the floor, or retreating from the lab group and reading her novel. As a reward for participating in lab group and for not falling to the floor, Sarah was allowed to go to the school library following class.

Related Instructional Targets for Social Communication: A Focus on Joint Attention Skills

An emerging body of research has focused on improving outcomes for students with ASD in the area of *joint attention*. Joint attention (JA) is defined as actively sharing and responding to a shared focus of attention with a communicative partner. Kasari and colleagues (Kasari, Paparella, Freeman, & Jahromi, 2008) distinguish *responsive joint attention,* where an individual follows a partner's gaze or point from *initiating joint attention,* in which an individual actively initiates sharing of interests and intentions. Even in advanced language users, social communication goals will likely focus on JA with the same inten-

sity and focus as other social communicative deficits, such as social-emotional reciprocity and/or perspective-taking ability. Perspective-taking considers partner's intentions based on both verbal and nonverbal cues, or modifying one's language in accordance with the agenda or perspective of a partner (Prizant, Wetherby, Rubin, & Rydell, 2006).

Beginning with joint attention (JA), the foundations of social reciprocity in early development are thought to be established before the child acquires conventional symbols, or language. Because it has been reported that up to 90% of children with ASD display deficits and delays in JA, it is a key skill to target as an intervention priority (Kasari et al., 2008). Interventions addressing JA have a measurable and early impact on infants, toddlers, and preschool-age children with ASD, many of whom might be considered to be at *pre-language* and *emerging language* stages of development. Establishment of JA at these two earliest communicative stages is critical, as this milestone is strongly predictive of later expressive language ability, and for some higher-functioning children, improved cognitive outcomes (Dawson et al., 2009; Kasari et al., 2008). Interventions facilitating JA in young children can make use of discrete trial teaching methods, where the child is prompted to follow a point from the adult, shift gaze to an object of focus, and is then reinforced for imitating a verbal model. They can also consist of naturalistic approaches, like PRT, where adults follow the child's lead in preferred activities and spontaneously imitate the child's communicative signals. Applied behavioral analysis methods combining discrete trial with naturalistic approaches have successfully established and increased the rate of JA as well as expressive language in children with ASD (Dawson et al., 2009; Kasari et al., 2008; Rogers et al., 2012; Whalen & Schreibman, 2003). Studies that have trained parents how to establish JA with their young children have yielded successful social communication outcomes for young children with ASD (Kasari et al., 2008; Patten & Watson, 2011; Siller, Hutman, & Sigman, 2013; Vernon, Koegel, Dauterman, & Stolen, 2012). Alternatively, some JA studies have utilized a model of mediated learning, in which parents of toddlers with ASD observe and learn principles of embedding nat-

ural turn-taking and JA routines with their children (Schertz, Odom, Baggett, & Sideris, 2012). The American Speech-Language-Hearing Association (ASHA, 2014) provides sample instructional JA goals at the prelinguistic, emerging, and advanced language stages of development that coaches and teachers can refer to when selecting goals to target in this area (Table 10–2).

Coaching Teachers in Social Reciprocity Instruction in Emerging Language Users

Emerging language users have progressed to a symbolic means of com-

Table 10–2. Sample Joint Attention Goals for Three Developmental Communication Stages

Prelanguage Stages	Emerging Language Stages	Advanced Language Stages
• Orienting toward people • Responding to a caregiver's voice • Shifting gaze between people and objects • Pairing gestures with gaze and/or physical contact to request and protest • Directing a partner's attention to an interesting item or event • Attending to emotional displays of distress • Sharing positive affect • Initiating social routines (e.g., peek-a-boo)	• Seeking specific emotional responses from others (e.g., comfort, showing off) • Commenting to share enjoyment and interests • Recognizing and describing emotional states of self and others	• Understanding what others are indicating with gaze and gestures • Determining causal factors for emotional states of self and others • Using emotions of others to guide behavior (e.g., selecting topics based on a partner's preferences, praising others) • Considering another's intentions and knowledge (e.g., requesting information from others, sharing information about past and future events)

Source: ASHA, 2014.

munication adopting speech and more conventional communicative gestures prevalent in the patterns of individuals around them. Developmental achievements in JA become more sophisticated for the child in this stage of language development. Nevertheless, it is common for discontinuities to exist between skill domains among students with ASD. For example, a student in advanced language stages with fluent conversational speech may demonstrate developmentally less advanced JA skills by failing to shift eye gaze responsively with partners in a communicative exchange (Prizant, Wetherby, Rubin, & Rydell, 2006). Because gaps in cognitive, linguistic, and social skill domains are common in ASD, it is essential that targeted skill areas for treatment not be selected in isolation of each other. This is especially true when social communication goals are the focus of instruction (ASHA, 2014). A case vignette for Ericka, a student with limited social reciprocity and JA, appears in Box 10–4.

An administrator of a comprehensive ASD program wanted to utilize an intensive and expert coaching model to support Ericka's IEP team, so she invited an HQC-A from the special education local agency to partner with the team. The coach had expertise in ASD and prior experience supporting teachers and therapists working with students with ASD. The coach made multiple visits to observe and video-record portions of Ericka's classroom day, noticing that her engagement and JA increased noticeably when simple turn-taking activities were presented to her. The coach helped the team reflect on this observation and facilitated conversation with the team to brainstorm activities where Ericka was regularly exposed to opportunities to initiate and respond to JA. This was achieved during her occupational therapy program and during snack, circle time, and break activities, where sharing of communicative intentions, physical proximity to a partner, and opportunities for shared positive affect were high. The coach further suggested an alternative to two-dimensional pictures that were so distracting for Ericka. An augmentative and alternative communication (AAC) application was loaded onto an electronic tablet device and was used to augment Ericka's communicative attempts and to allow her to rehearse speech output from the device. The IEP team and coach felt that this would resolve her distractibility with paper (two-dimensional) visual supports. The coach then asked the team to brainstorm where the tablet could be meaningfully embedded into routine activities of the day. One of Ericka's revised communication IEP goals was to participate in reciprocal turn-taking exchanges with partners, and to increase her rate of responding appropriately to "what" and "where" questions (e.g., "What does Ericka want?"; "Where does Ericka go?"). The team decided that Ericka should have ready access to her tablet at all circle, recess, and snack activities where opportunities for making requests were frequent. Ericka could also be prompted to respond to questions about an ongoing activity (e.g., "What day is it?"; 'What's the weather?') using the tablet.

Initially, Ericka required extensive support to point accurately to items pictured on her tablet. Because

---

Box 10–4. Vignette: Ericka

Ericka was a 5-year-old with moderate to severe ASD. She had a small repertoire of single words used to make various requests ("potty," "water," "candy," "snack," "more"). However, her rate of spontaneous bids for interaction with adults in the classroom was extremely low, and she did not seem to notice or interact with peers. By parent report, Ericka's two-word speech was just emerging at home, although her rate of communication attempts at school was low. During circle time, she was rarely responsive to communicative bids from the teacher or behavioral aide. When group songs were introduced and noise levels increased, Ericka reacted by plugging her ears with her fingers and fleeing from the activity. On one occasion, she repeatedly verbalized a request: "Go home."

Attempts at augmenting Ericka's communication with picture symbols were met with failure because of her pattern of grabbing and repetitively flicking any paper material (photos, art materials, magazines, picture books) near her face. Even an electronic AAC device with picture overlays that displayed vocabulary items on 8 × 11-inch paper was distracting; she pulled out the picture overlays and flapped them. The team SLP and teacher sought consultative coaching support from the special education agency's HQC-A to problem solve ways to circumvent this repetitive motor behavior that was disruptive to Ericka's social and communicative progress.

---

her fine-motor control was a problem, her occupational therapist found that a pointing stylus was beneficial to help her isolate the images on the tablet. Over the course of the summer, Ericka made steady progress with requesting in naturally occurring communication contexts. A videotape of her communicative turns, including her responsive and initiating JA at baseline and 6 months after intervention was collected. In post-baseline sessions with prompting from her aide, Ericka selected snack food choices when asked what she wanted to eat. She also responded to a question about the day of the week ("It's Tuesday"). Although she was not using the device to initiate spontaneous communicative bids with peers, the coach and IEP team noted that her rate of verbal requests had increased from baseline. Additionally, Ericka was beginning to show increased shared attention with adults (e.g., approaching her instructional assistant in turn-taking activities with action toys, and greeting the coach at recess and class time).

Coaching Social Communication Instruction to Address Social Skills

The comprehensive and specific EBIs reviewed thus far have direct application to the social skill needs of students with ASD, and it is worth discussing these skills a bit further. As applied research addressing social communication treatments has increased, focused interventions targeting students with more sophisticated language have examined what instructional elements seem to have the greatest impact on social skills. Well-controlled studies point to small but significant results in teaching some aspect of social interaction or social knowledge (Burgess & Turkstra, 2006; McConnell, 2002). However, favorable outcomes are variable depending on the (a) social behavior symptoms of the individuals with ASD; (b) the social skills targeted; (c) the intervention approaches used and their degree of naturalness; (d) whether interventions involve group or individual teaching; and (e) the assessments used to evaluate social skills improvement (Williams-White, Keonig, & Scahill, 2007). Some studies point to the need to match a particular type of social skill deficit with an

intervention specifically targeted to it, and a need for determining the dose of social skills training for generalization of skills to take place (Bellini, Peters, Benner, & Hopf, 2007).

Although there are burgeoning resources on the educational market that target some aspect of social skill improvement, Williams-White et al. (2007) cautioned that there is "no standardized, manual-based curricula for social skills training designed for students with ASDs." There are, however, general goals for improving social skills that have merit. Williams-White and colleagues break these down into four broad skill objectives: (a) increasing the rate of social initiations, (b) improving social responding, (c) reducing interfering behaviors, and (d) promoting skills generalization (Williams-White et al., 2007). Examples of supportive strategies are further detailed in Table 10–3.

Summary

Social communication is a critical skill domain to target at all skill levels in individuals with ASD. A suggested route to coaching the instruction of these skills begins with educational best practices emphasizing the importance of spontaneous communication in natural social contexts with opportunities for peer interaction. In addition, teachers and teams need to consider family priorities to construct relevant IEP goals for students challenged by core deficits in social communication across the life span of individuals with this disorder.

Table 10–3. Goals and Supportive Social Communication Strategies in Advanced Symbol Users

Increase Social Initiations	Increase Social Responding	Reduce Interfering Behavior	Promote Skills Generalization
Make social rules clear and concrete (e.g., "stand an arm's length away from your partner")	Teach social response scripts (e.g., answering personal information questions)	Review socially appropriate and inappropriate behaviors of participants in the social group (e.g., no full-body hugging)	Use multiple individuals and trainers to transfer skills Involve parents/family in the training steps
Model age-appropriate social initiation strategies (greetings, making "small talk")	Model and role-play to teach and practice responsiveness	Differentially reinforce prosocial behaviors	Make teaching predictable, engaging. and developmentally relevant
Use natural motivation for social initiations (e.g., following a partner's conversational lead and interests)	Reinforce response attempts	Allow students to chart their own behavior	Practice skills taught in natural settings (e.g., lunchroom, hallways, recess, community settings, home)

Source: Adapted from Williams-White et al., 2007.

End-of-Chapter Questions

1. As an HQC-A, what variables would be important to consider in coaching a team as they draft IEP goals for social communication?

2. Using the sequence of components in a single discrete instructional trial, as outlined in Figure 10–1, create an example of a single trial for an instructional target of your choice. Be sure to provide examples for how each component will be implemented.

3. Provide an example of an instructional trial utilizing a PRT approach that incorporates each of the four strategies identified in this chapter for capturing the pivotal area of student motivation (child choice, direct and natural reinforcers, interspersing maintenance trials, and reinforcing attempts).

4. When teaching social communication skills, what student and treatment variables might dictate outcomes when working with students diagnosed with ASD?

5. What is a social narrative? What value does this intervention have with advanced language users?

6. Describe one or more social communication interventions that you could effectively coach with an IEP team serving teens having difficulty reading nonverbal social cues.

References

American Psychiatric Association. (2013). *Diagnostic and statistical manual of mental disorders* (5th ed.). Washington, DC: Author.

American Speech-Language-Hearing Association. (2014). *Sample intervention goals based on core challenges in autism spectrum disorder.* Retrieved July 27, 2015, from http://www.asha.org/uploadedFiles/ASHA/Practice_Portal/Clinical_Topics/Autism/Sample%20Intervention%20Goals.pdf

Barahav, E., & Darling, R. (2007). Case report: Using an auditory trainer with caregiver video modeling to enhance communication and socialization behaviors in autism. *Journal of Autism and Developmental Disorders, 38*(4), 771–775.

Bellini, S., & Akullian, J. (2007). A meta-analysis of video modeling and self modeling interventions for children and adolescent with autism spectrum disorders. *Exceptional Children, 73*(3), 264–287.

Bellini, S., Peters, J. K., Benner, L., & Hopf, A. (2007). A meta-analysis of school-based social skills interventions for children with autism spectrum disorders. *Remedial and Special Education, 28*(3), 153–162.

Burgess, S., & Turkstra, L. S. (2006). Social skills intervention for adolescents with autism spectrum disorders: A review of the experimental evidence. *EPB Briefs, 1*(4), 1–16.

Chan, J., Lang, R., Rispoli, M., O'Reilly, M., Sigafoos, J., & Cole, H. (2009). Use of peer-mediated interventions in the treatment of autism spectrum disorders: A systematic review. *Research in Autism Spectrum Disorders, 3*, 876–889.

Charlop, M., & Milstein, J. (1989). Teaching autistic children conversational speech using video modeling. *Journal of Applied Behavior Analysis, 22*(3), 275–285.

Collet-Klingenberg, L., & Franzone, E. (2008). *Overview of social narratives.* Madison, WI: The National Professional Development Center on Autism Spectrum Disorders, Waisman Center, University of Wisconsin.

Corbett, B. A., & Abdullah, M. (2005). Video modeling: Why does it work for children with autism? *Journal of Early and Intensive Behavior Intervention, 2*(1), 2–8.

Dawson, G., Rogers, S., Munson, J., Smith, M., Winter, J., Greenson, J., . . . Varley, J. (2009). Randomized, controlled trial of an intervention for toddlers with autism: The Early Start Denver Model. *Pediatrics, 125*(1), e17–e23.

Dollaghan, C., & Kaston, N. (1986). A comprehension monitoring program for language-impaired children. *Journal of Speech and Hearing Disorders, 51*, 264–271.

Garcia-Albea, E., Reeve, S. A., Brothers, K. J., & Reeve, K. F. (2014). Using audio script fading and multiple-exemplar training to increase vocal interactions in children with autism. *Journal of Applied Behavior Analysis, 47*(2), 325–343.

Goldstein, H., Schneider, N., & Thiemann, K. (2007). Peer-mediated social communication intervention: When clinical expertise informs treatment development and evaluation. *Topics in Language Disorders*, *27*, 182–199.

Gray, C. (2010). *The new social story book.* Arlington, TX: Future Horizons.

Gray, C., & Garand, J. D. (1993). Social Stories: Improving responses of students with autism with accurate social information. *Focus on Autistic Behavior*, *8*(1), 1–10.

Gray, C., & White, A. L. (2002). *My Social Stories book.* London, UK: Jessica Kingsley.

Kamps, D., Thiemann-Bourque, K., Heitzman-Powell, L., Schwartz, I., Rosenberg, N., Mason, R., & Cox, S. (2015). A comprehensive peer network intervention to improve social communication of children with autism spectrum disorders: A randomized trial in kindergarten and first grade. *Journal of Autism and Developmental Disorders*, *45*(6), 1809–1824.

Karhaneh, M., Clark, B., Ospina, M. B., Selda, J. C., Smith, V., & Hartling, L. (2010). Social Stories™ to improve social skills in children with autism spectrum disorder: A systematic review. *Autism*, *14*(6), 641–662.

Kasari, C., Paparella, T., Freeman, S., & Jahromi, L. B. (2008). Language outcome in autism: Randomized comparison of joint attention and play interventions. *Journal of Consultative and Clinical Psychology*, *76*(1), 125–137.

Kasari, C., & Patterson, S. (2012). Interventions addressing social impairments in autism. *Current Psychiatry Reports*, *14*(6), 713–725.

Koegel, L. K., Koegel, R. L., Harrower, J. K., & Carter, C. M. (1999). Pivotal response intervention I: Overview of approach. *Journal of the Association for Persons with Severe Handicaps*, *24*(3), 174–185.

Koegel, L. K., Park, M. N., & Koegel, R. L. (2014). Using self-management to improve the reciprocal social conversation of children with autism spectrum disorder. *Journal of Autism and Developmental Disorders*, *44*(5), 1055–1063.

Koegel, R. L., & Frea, W. D. (1993). Treatment of social behavior in autism through the modification of pivotal social skills. *Journal of Applied Behavior Analysis*, *26*(3), 369–377.

Koegel, R. L., & Koegel, L. K. (2006). *Pivotal response treatments for autism: Communication, social, and academic development.* Baltimore, MD: Paul H. Brookes.

Koegel, R. L., & Koegel, L. K. (2012). *The PRT pocket guide: Pivotal response treatment for autism spectrum disorder.* Baltimore, MD: Paul H. Brookes.

Koegel, R. L., O'Dell, M. C., & Koegel, L. K. (1987). A natural language teaching paradigm for nonverbal autistic children. *Journal of Autism and Developmental Disorders*, *17*(2), 187–200.

Krantz, P. J., & McClannahan, L. E. (1998). Social interaction skills for children with autism: A script-fading procedure for beginning readers. *Journal of Applied Behavior Analysis*, *31*(2), 191–202.

Maione, L., & Mirenda, P. (2006). Effects of video modeling and video feedback on peer-directed social language skills of a child with autism. *Journal of Positive Behavior Interventions*, *8*(2), 106–118.

McConnell, S. R. (2002). Interventions to facilitate social interaction for young children with autism: Review of available research and recommendations for educational intervention and future research. *Journal of Autism and Developmental Disorders*, *32*(5), 351–372.

Merrison, S., & Merrison, A. J. (2005). Repair in speech and language therapy interaction: Investigating pragmatic language impairment of children. *Child Language Teaching and Therapy*, *212*, 191–211.

National Autism Center. (2015). *Findings and conclusions: National standards project, phase 2.* Randolph, MA: Author.

Nikopoulos, C., & Nikopoulou-Smyrni, P. (2008). Teaching complex social skills to children with autism: Advances of video modeling. *Journal of Early and Intensive Behavior Intervention*, *5*(2), 30–43.

Paterson, C., & Arco, L. (2007). Using video modeling for generalizing toy play in children with autism. *Behavior Modification*, *31*(5), 660–681.

Patten, E., & Watson, L. R. (2011). Interventions targeting attention in young children with autism. *American Journal Speech-Language Pathology*, *20*, 60–69.

Pierce, K., & Schreibman, L. (1995). Increasing complex social behaviors in children with autism: Effects of peer-implemented pivotal response training. *Journal of Applied Behavior Analysis*, *28*(3), 285–295.

Pierce, K., & Schreibman, L. (1997). Multiple peer use of pivotal response training to increase social behaviors of classmates with autism: Results from trained and untrained peers. *Journal of Applied Behavior Analysis*, *30*(1), 157–160.

Prizant, B., Wetherby, A. M., Rubin, E., & Rydell, P. (2006). *The SCERTS Model program planning and intervention: A comprehensive educational approach for young children with autism spectrum disorders, Volume 2: Program planning and intervention*. Baltimore, MD: Brookes.

Rogers, S. J., & Dawson, G. (2009). *Play and engagement in early autism: The Early Start Denver Model. Volume I: The treatment*. New York, NY: Guilford Press.

Rogers, S. J., Dawson, G., & Vismara, L. A. (2012). *An early start for your child with autism: Using everyday activities to help kids connect, communicate, and learn. proven methods based on the breakthrough Early Start Denver Model*. New York, NY: Guilford Press.

Rogers, S. J., Estes, A., Lord, C., Vismara, L., Winter, J., Fitzpatrick, A., & Dawson, G. (2012). Effects of a Brief Early Start Denver Model (ESDM)–based parent intervention on toddlers at risk for autism spectrum disorders: A randomized controlled trial. *Journal of the American Academy of Child & Adolescent Psychiatry*, *51*, 1052–1065.

Sarokoff, R. A., Taylor, B. A., & Poulson, C. L. (2001). Teaching children with autism to engage in conversational exchanges: Script fading with embedded textual stimuli. *Journal of Applied Behavior Analysis*, *34*(1), 81–84.

Schertz, H., Odom, S. L., Bagget, K. M., & Sideris, H. H. (2012). Effects of joint attention mediated learning for toddlers with autism spectrum disorders: An initial randomized controlled study. *Early Childhood Research Quarterly*, *28*, 249–258.

Siller, M., Hutman, T., & Sigman, M. (2013). A parent-mediated intervention to increase responsive parental behaviors and child communication in children with autism spectrum disorder: A randomized clinical trial. *Journal of Autism and Developmental Disorders*, *43*(3), 540–555.

Smith, T. (2001). Discrete trial training in the treatment of autism. *Focus on Autism and Other Developmental Disabilities*, *16*(2), 86–92.

Thiemann, K. S., & Goldstein, H. (2004). Effects of peer training and written text cueing on social communication of school-age children with pervasive developmental disorder. *Journal of Speech, Language, and Hearing Research*, *47*, 126–144.

Thiemann-Bourque, K. S. (2010). Navigating the transition to middle school: Peer network programming for students with autism spectrum disorder. *The ASHA Leader*, *15*, 12–15.

Vernon, T. W., Koegel, R. L., Dauterman, H., & Stolen, K. (2012). An early social engagement intervention for young children with autism and their parents. *Journal of Autism and Developmental Disorders*, *42*, 2702–2717.

Whalen, C., & Schreibman, L. (2003). Joint attention training for children with autism using behavior modification procedures. *Journal of Child Psychology and Psychiatry, 44*(3), 456–468.

Williams-White, S., Keonig, K., & Scahill, L. (2007). Social skills development in children with autism spectrum disorders: A review of the intervention research. *Journal of Autism and Developmental Disorders, 37,* 1858–1868.

Wolfberg, P. J., & Schuler, A. L. (1993). Integrated playgroups: A model for promoting the social and cognitive dimensions of play in children with autism. *Journal of Autism and Developmental Disorders, 23*(3), 467–489.

Wong, C., Odom, S. L., Hume, K., Cox, A. W., Fettig, A., Kucharczyk, S., . . . Schultz, T. R. (2014). *Evidence-based practices for children, youth, and young adults with Autism Spectrum Disorder.* Chapel Hill, NC: The University of North Carolina, Frank Porter Graham Child Development Institute, Autism Evidence-Based Practice Review Group.

Woods, J. J., & Wetherby, A. M. (2003). Early identification of and intervention for infants and toddlers who are at risk for autism spectrum disorder. *Language, Speech, and Hearing Services in Schools, 34*(3), 180–193.

CHAPTER 11

Using High-Quality Coaching to Support Teachers in Addressing Behavioral Issues for Students With ASD

We can't solve problems by using the same kind of thinking we used when we created them.

—Albert Einstein

Chapter Objectives

■ Review the primary reasons to prioritize behavior, interests, and activity selection for students with autism spectrum disorder (ASD).

■ Highlight identified evidence-based interventions that address behavior and expand the range of interests and activities among individuals on the autism spectrum.

■ Demonstrate how high-quality coaching can enhance the ability of teachers to effectively intervene with student challenging behaviors and in expanding the range of interests and activities for students with ASD.

Rationale: Why Focus on Behavior?

In addition to difficulties in the area of social communication, individuals with ASD often display what has been referred to as "restricted, repetitive patterns of behavior, interests or activities" (APA, 2013), as was discussed in Chapter 2. As seen in the vignette in Box 11–1, restricted or repetitive behaviors, interests, and activities among students with ASD can pose particular challenges in school settings, where these behaviors can result in increased anxiety for the student due to increased exposure to transitions, changes in routine, and sensory experiences. Furthermore, these restricted or repetitive behaviors, interests, and activities may result in the student with ASD being isolated from or even ostracized by peers. Therefore, it is critical that coaches and teachers work together to provide positive and effective behavioral and social supports to students in these areas. Fortunately, a great deal of research has demonstrated the effectiveness of addressing challenging behaviors, expanding the range of interests, and increasing engagement in a range of activities among students with ASD. Furthermore, an increasing number of useful resources to support coaches and teachers in this area are being made available, such as those provided in Chapter 9 (see Box 9–1). The remainder of this chapter will review evidence-based practices, identify resources, and provide guidelines for providing high-quality coaching with teachers seeking to address the restrictive, repetitive behaviors, interests, and activities of students with ASD.

Box 11–1. Vignette: Coaching Needed

Elias was just hired to take on a middle school ASD program in the middle of the year. Elias had been a long-term substitute at the school for the fall semester in a seventh-grade social studies class. He had obtained his teaching credential in English a few years back but was unable to find a job close by and wanted to stay in the area. The principal liked his youthful exuberance when interacting with students on campus. He was personable, approachable, and the students seemed to enjoy his offbeat but effective teaching style. The school had run through three special education teachers in the past 2 years, and now the third had quit right after the bell rang on the last day of the fall semester. The self-contained program for students with ASD was notorious for loud outbursts and students running out of the classroom, and instruction was inconsistent at best. The class was well staffed with two behavior technicians, two instructional assistants, and one teacher for 12 students; however, several of the students had significant behavioral challenges and social skill deficits with which former teachers and instructional assistants could not deal with successfully. So the principal reasoned: Why not hire someone who has the right attitude to take over the class that had caused him much consternation over the last 2½ years? Because Elias held a credential in general education, the principal thought that with some coursework in special education and with some intensive coaching, he could handle the job. The principal called up the director of special education and offered her a deal: "I hire Elias in this very troubled class, and you hire a coach from Able Train, a well-respected agency that provides support for professionals working with students with ASD." He then posed a second part of the deal; the coach would have to be there 5 days a week for the next 3 weeks and then taper to 3 days for 2 weeks, paring down to two, or fewer visits over the next month, and eventually moving to a consultative coaching approach for the remainder of the semester. If need be, the coach could move back to an intensive coaching arrangement to ensure Elias' success.

The principal was committed to support Elias at every turn but needed the extra support from a well-trained and knowledgeable coach with expertise in evidence-based practices for students with ASD who would be there for Elias throughout his maiden voyage into the world of special education, as well as dealing with a tough assignment. The special education director had just received some flow-through dollars from the federal government and decided that a good use of some of the extra money should be allocated to this class, so the director agreed to hire the coach from Able Train to provide intensive guidance for Elias.

Review of Evidence-Based Interventions for Supporting the Behavior of Students With ASD

Research has overwhelmingly established the effectiveness of techniques derived from the field of applied behavior analysis in successfully addressing a wide range of challenging behaviors, as well as in promoting a host of appropriate, prosocial behaviors. For example, the National Professional Development Center published a comprehensive review of the research and identified 27 interventions as evidence-based practices (EBPs) for individuals with ASD (Wong et al., 2014). Additionally, the National Standards Project published a similar comprehensive review, identifying 14 practices as "Established Interventions" and 18 as "Promising Interventions" (National Autism Center, 2015). The discrepancy in numbers between the two reports is primarily due to how individual interventions were grouped into categories by each project, but the bottom line is that coaches and teachers currently have an array of EBPs to draw from in addressing the behaviors of students with ASD. The current issue facing coaches and teachers then is one of selecting the right EBP for the right situation, and ensuring proficient application to accurately implement a range of EBPs to address the restricted, repetitive behaviors, interests, and activities among their students. Each of the following sections provides resources, guidelines, and information for coaches

and teachers to support the pursuit of this goal.

Addressing Student Challenging Behavior

When it comes to addressing challenging behavior, there are multiple levels of support that schools and teachers can provide to implement various EBPs. Recently, many schools and districts have undertaken school-wide reform efforts to more effectively support the behavior of all students in a school. Multitiered systems of behavioral support, such as Positive Behavior Interventions and Support (PBIS), consist of the implementation of behavior support systems that increase with intensity to match the level of support needed by students (i.e., universal, targeted, and individualized intervention systems). Thus, the level of supports implemented for all students are of relatively low intensity and tend to address the behavioral needs of most students. Universal behavior supports consist of establishing school-wide expectations, teaching these expectations to all students, establishing practices for acknowledging students when they meet expectations, developing clear and consistent procedures for responding to challenging behavior, and using data on challenging behavior to identify patterns and make decisions on changes to behavior supports. However, some students will require additional supports, which must increase in their intensity to address these needs. These targeted behavior supports tend to be group-oriented interventions and consist of increasing the explicit instruction of behavior expectations, and providing opportunities for reinforcement and monitoring of student progress. A few students will require highly intensive and individualized behavior supports to effectively address the level of behavioral need they display. Interventions at this individualized level of support are characterized by function-based behavior support plans developed by a team of individuals supporting the student in question (Sugai et al., 2000). The implications of these multitiered systems of behavior supports for students with ASD and their teachers are many. Positive Behavior Intervention Support provides a common language for all educators, administrators, and related support personnel to converse about and problem solve issues related to student challenging behavior, potentially increasing consistency with behavior support plan implementation for students with ASD. The establishment of school-wide behavior supports for all students, students at-risk for challenging behavior, and students with chronic challenging behavior can improve outcomes, including those receiving special education services (Tobin, Horner, Vincent, & Swain-Bradway, 2012). Thus, having school-wide behavioral supports in place allows special education and related services personnel to focus on supporting those students with the most intensive behavioral needs. Although traditional views on behavior support for students with ASD would be characterized as occurring exclusively at the intensive, individualized, function-

based behavior support planning level, multiple levels of behavior support (of lesser intensity) can also be of benefit. Coaches can support teachers by utilizing the framework provided by PBIS to ensure the design and implementation of comprehensive behavior supports for students with ASD.

Using HQC-A to Support Teachers in Addressing the Behavior of Students With ASD

Positive Behavior Interventions and Support provides a useful framework for coaches and teachers in designing and implementing comprehensive classroom systems of behavior support for students with ASD. In designing behavioral systems, coaches and teachers work together to establish each of the following levels of PBIS for their students: (a) universal supports that would be made available to all; (b) targeted, group-oriented supports for those who share common behavioral needs (e.g., social skills, transitioning, etc.); and (c) intensive, individualized function-based behavior supports for students with chronic and challenging behavior. As each of these levels are characterized by an increasing level of intensity in terms of planning, implementation, and monitoring, they map nicely with the levels of intensity characterized in high-quality coaching. With peer-to-peer coaching (PtP) being of relatively low intensity, this approach may function ideally in the development and implementation of universal behavior supports for all students with ASD. Likewise, consultative coaching (CC) consists of an increase in coaching intensity, and as such lends itself well to the development and implementation of targeted behavior supports. Last, intensive coaching (IC), as the most intensive level of support in the HQC-A model, is ideally suited for teachers who need to implement individualized levels of behavior support. It should be noted, however, that these coaching levels are not restricted to the levels of behavior support indicated above. For instance, a given teacher may be well versed in delivering the individualized level of PBIS, and perhaps would benefit from a colleague (peer) providing informal feedback on a drafted functional assessment and behavior support plan, prior to its implementation in the classroom. Likewise, some teachers may struggle with effectively implementing universal PBIS (e.g., classroom management), and require a more intensive level of coaching support than would be available with PtP coaching. The following chapter sections provide guidelines for educators and coaches who work with students on the autism spectrum in increasing the level of coaching support provided to teachers as the levels of behavior support also increase in intensity.

Universal Behavior Supports for Students With ASD: Addressed With Peer-to-Peer Coaching

One of the areas in which many teachers struggle is in the implementation of effective classroom management practices designed to address the behavioral needs of all students (Pas, Bradshaw, Hershfeldt, & Leaf, 2010). This can certainly also be the case for teachers who instruct individuals with ASD. It is important here to note that students with ASD are served in a variety of classroom arrangements. Many are fully included with special education supports being provided in general education grade-level classrooms where they participate with their typically developing peers. Others receive services in self-contained settings for either part or all of their school day. Still others attend self-contained programs exclusive to ASD. Although the logistics for delivering behavior supports in the variety of educational settings in which students with ASD participate will vary, the approaches that are described in this chapter are appropriate for any type of educational setting. And even though classroom management can be a struggle for many teachers, much is known about establishing effective class-wide systems of behavior support for all. Furthermore, much of this information is publicly available in user-friendly formats specifically designed for teachers (Table 11–1). Peer-to-peer (PtP) coaching can be an effective way of supporting teachers who struggle in this area.

Classroom Rules and Procedures. One of the first areas to address in the development of an effective class-wide behavior support system is the establishment of classroom rules and procedures. *Rules* can be defined as guidelines for expected student behavior that cut

Table 11–1. Online Resources on Classroom Management

Resources	Location
American Psychological Association's Classroom Management Modules	http://www.apa.org/ed/schools/cpse/activities/class-management.aspx
IRIS Star Legacy Modules Classroom Management (Part 1): Learning the Components of a Comprehensive Behavior Management Plan Classroom Management (Part 2): Developing Your Own Comprehensive Behavior Management Plan	http://iris.peabody.vanderbilt.edu/

across all classroom (or even school) activities. On the other hand, *procedures* refer to the specific steps students are expected to follow within a targeted routine or activity. Thus, rules tend to be more broadly stated, encompassing broader concepts of behavior for which specific examples and nonexamples will need to be provided in order to clarify the concept. Rules should be positively stated in order to focus student (and teacher) attention on what behaviors are expected. They should be limited in number to no more than three to five rules, so that all students could be expected to memorize them. Examples of rules include "Be Respectful," "Be Responsible," "Be Safe," and so on. If the school is implementing school-wide PBIS, they will have established school-wide behavior expectations. Although general education teachers are commonly expected to incorporate these school-wide expectations as the class-room rules, and provide examples contextualizing how those school-wide expectations manifest themselves in the classroom setting (e.g., "In the classroom the school expectation 'Be Respectful' means raising your hand before speaking"). Sometimes, special educators serving students in self-contained classroom settings may feel the need to maintain their own classroom rules separate from the school-wide expectations; however, this may be a missed opportunity for programs serving students with ASD to participate in the broader general education school culture. Additionally, by adopting broader school-wide expectations as the class rules, and teaching students with ASD what those labels mean in the classroom, the prompting and reinforcement provided across adult partners and settings can promote generalization of that skill to new settings on campus (e.g., cafeteria, hallway, general education classrooms, etc.).

Directly related to the establishment of rules and procedures is the practice of providing direct and explicit instruction of these rules and expectations. In order for students to learn the associations between the terms identified in the classroom rules and corresponding expected behaviors, direct instruction related to the class rules will need to be provided. General guidelines for teaching classroom rules are outlined in Table 11–2.

Each of the steps identified in Table 11–2 is essential to teaching classroom rules if we want students to demonstrate the expected behaviors. Teachers in a PtP coaching arrangement can support each other by collaborating on the development of lesson plans to teach common classroom rules. Table 11–3 shows an example of a lesson plan for teaching the classroom rule, "Be Respectful."

Table 11–4 provides a template that can be used as a guide in the development of lesson plans for additional classroom rules. The PtP coaches, teachers, and other classroom staff can work together during planning time to develop common lesson plans to be shared in multiple classrooms, and can divide up the responsibility of developing lesson plans. Following up after lesson plan delivery to revise, update, and provide feedback to each other can enhance the effectiveness of this PtP coaching process.

Whereas classroom rules identify behaviors that students are expected to display across all activities, procedures are step-by-step guidelines expected of students in order to successfully participate in a specific activity. Like rules, procedures should be positively stated and limited in number to three to five per activity. Thus, procedures are aligned with specific routines or activities and, in a sense function as examples of how the class rules are manifested within these routines/activities. When planning to teach procedures, it is particularly helpful for coaches and teachers to conduct a task analysis (see Chapter 8) of the targeted routine/activity, in order to identify the critical steps. Subsequently, those steps that students have

Table 11–2. Guidelines for Teaching Rules

1. Select rule to teach.

2. Define and list the critical attributes of selected rule.

3. Provide examples and nonexamples of rule.

4. Develop activities to enhance student understanding of the rule.

5. Develop activities to check for student understanding of the rule.

6. Develop activities to extend student understanding of the rule to new areas of application

Table 11–3. Sample Lesson Plan for Teaching Rule "Be Respectful"

Rule Targeted: Be Respectful
Definition and Critical Attributes: To show concern or consideration: Behaviors that help people feel calmer, safer, friendlier, and more cooperative

Examples:	**Nonexamples:**
Listen during lessons Hold the door open Ask before touching things that belong to others	Grab materials Call people names Make noises during lessons

Activities to Enhance Concept Development: Have students write and then share and role-play examples that they developed for what being respectful looks like.
Activities to Check for Understanding: Present examples and nonexamples. Have students identify the examples. Examples and nonexamples can be presented in pictures or in writing.
Activities to Extend Concept Development: Assign topics for journal entries related to the concept. Ask students to keep frequency counts of examples and nonexamples observed in a television program. Graph the results.

particular difficulty with can be selected as the primary focus of instruction when teaching the procedures for the identified routine/activity.

Once procedures have been identified for targeted activities, they also must be directly taught to students. Table 11–5 provides a sample Lesson

Table 11–4. Lesson Plan for Teaching Rules

Rule Targeted:	
Definition and Critical Attributes:	
Examples:	**Nonexamples:**
Activities to Enhance Concept Development:	
Activities to Check for Understanding:	
Activities to Extend Concept Development:	

Plan for teaching procedures for a classroom transition routine.

When teaching procedures, it is important to review the class rules and to draw connections for students with ASD between the procedural steps and the rules they exemplify. Examples and nonexamples for each procedural step being taught should then be identified to provide opportunities for students to discriminate between the two when the lesson is presented. The next step in teaching procedures is to provide opportunities for students to practice.

Table 11–5. Lesson Plan for Teaching Procedure "Transition to Circle"

Setting: Classroom		
List Rules (List those that apply to selected routine/activity): A. Be Respectful B. Be Prepared C. Follow Directions D. E.	**Activity for Reviewing Rules:**	
Generate Specific Procedures for Routine/Activity		
Target Activity: Transition to group circle activity		
Procedure (related Rule):	**Example**	**Nonexample**
a. Put away materials when timer beeps (Follow Directions)	a. Student places book on bookshelf	a. Student continues looking at book
b. Walk quietly to circle area (Be Respectful)	b. Student walks to circle	b. Student skips on tip toes to circle
c. Sit on tape border of circle, criss-cross applesauce (Be Prepared)	c. Student sits on tape with legs crossed	c. Student sits in middle of circle
d.	d.	d.

continues

Table 11–5. *continued*

Activities to Allow Students to Practice Desired Behaviors:
Hold a group circle activity where a highly preferred snack will be provided. When the timer beeps, students will be physically prompted using a least-to-most prompting sequence to put materials away, walk quietly to the circle, and sit with legs crossed on the tape border of the circle area. Any challenging behaviors/refusals to transition will be corrected by reinitiating the transition sequence from the beginning.

Plan for Recognizing Appropriate Behavior:
Once students have correctly followed the procedural steps, they will be provided with a snack. Behavior-specific praise will be provided following student completion of each procedural step (e.g., "nice job putting away the paper!").

The practice activity should take place in the same location, with the same people and under the same conditions in which the targeted routine/activity would typically occur. However, the practice activity should intentionally be designed to be highly preferred and of low effort so that the only student demands related to acquisition skills are the procedural steps themselves. Last, a plan for reinforcing students when they follow each of the procedural steps and when they complete the routine successfully should be implemented. As with the development of class rules, coaches, and teachers in a PtP coaching arrangement can collaborate on the development and delivery of lesson plans for teaching the procedures for various routines and activities. The Lesson Plan for Teaching Procedures shown in Table 11–6 can be used as a template for this work.

Table 11–6. Lesson Plan for Teaching Procedures

Setting:		
List Rules (Circle those that apply to selected setting):	**Activity for Reviewing Rules:**	
A.		
B.		
C.		
D.		
E.		

Generate Specific Procedures for Routine/Activity

Target Activity:

Procedure (related Rule):	Example	Nonexample
a.	a.	a.
b.	b.	b.
c.	c.	c.
d.	d.	d.

continues

Table 11–6. *continued*

Activities to Allow Students to Practice Desired Behaviors:

Plan for Recognizing Appropriate Behavior:

Class-Wide Reinforcement Systems. Another foundational practice in effective behavior support is the establishment and active use of a class-wide incentive system to reinforce appropriate student behavior. *Reinforcement* can be defined as any event that follows a target behavior (added or taken away) that increases the likelihood that the same behavior will occur again in the future (Cooper, Heron, & Heward, 2007). Hence, when implementing a reinforcement system, the coach and teacher must engage in preference assessment activities to identify potential reinforcers to provide contingently when students display desired appropriate behaviors. Praise can be a particularly effective reinforcer, especially when praise specifies the desired behavior (Simonsen et al., 2008). For some students, however, praise may not function as reinforcement. In these cases, it should be paired with other events that do function as reinforcers, so that through this pairing it can take on reinforcing properties over time.

One of the more practical and effective class-wide incentive systems is token economy. A token economy involves contingently providing tokens, chips, stickers, check marks, points, or other items/markings to students who demonstrate desired behaviors identified by the teachers. Students may periodically exchange the tokens for other items, hypothesized by the teacher to function as reinforcers. Thus, through

stimulus pairing, tokens themselves can take on conditioned reinforcing properties, strengthening desirable student behavior. Table 11–7 presents the steps for setting up a token economy system, and coaches can support teachers with resources, examples, and feedback in the development of these systems to serve students with ASD. A variation on the token economy that allows for further individualization for students is the use of token boards. Despite the name, token boards are typically laminated sheets of paper, cardboard, or particle-board displaying a table of empty boxes. Teachers or classroom staff can then make marks in the boxes using dry erase markers, with each mark functioning like a token in that the adult shows the student the mark being made and

Table 11–7. Guidelines for Establishing a Token Economy

1. Select behaviors to be reinforced.
2. State desired behaviors in specific and observable terms.
3. Decide how you will measure the behaviors.
4. Decide where to monitor the behaviors.
5. Select the token.
6. Select your back-up reinforcers.
7. Place a value on the tokens.
8. Finalize the details by developing your own monitoring sheet to keep track of awards, and decide how often and when tokens can be exchanged for reinforcers.
9. Start your program.
10. Periodically modify your system to wean your students from the token economy.

delivers behavior specific praise. Once the boxes are filled with marks, the student can be given access to a backup reinforcer (e.g., edible, preferred activity, etc.).

Error Correction. In addition to teaching the class rules and procedures, providing opportunities for students to practice those rules and procedures for which they are appropriately reinforced, teachers also need to develop error correction strategies in order to respond appropriately when challenging behavior does occur. Error correction involves treating problem behavior as an incorrect response, or "error," and providing instruction and/or increasing assistance to enhance the student's capacity to respond to the circumstance (with a more desirable behavior). The first step with error correction is to intervene to prevent, or stop the performance of the "error" (i.e., problem behavior). The second step is to recreate or reestablish the context in which the "correct" performance should occur (e.g., reinitiate a transition routine). Last, provide another opportunity for the student to perform the correct behavior; delivering sufficient assistance, followed immediately with reinforcement paired with behavior specific praise for any reasonable attempt made by the student.

Daily Schedules. As discussed previously, many students with ASD find changes in routine and transitions from one activity to another to be particularly challenging. Given the prevalence of this issue for students with ASD, an effective

class-wide practice is to develop clear and accessible visual supports (Wong et al., 2014). For many students with ASD, providing a daily schedule in a picture format and teaching the procedures for schedule following can be extremely beneficial (National Autism Center, 2015). A schedule is used to identify the activities to be completed and the order in which they should be completed (Cohen & Sloan, 2007). Although many formats can be used for a daily schedule, the use of pictures or icons to represent each major activity of the day can enhance the students' ability to make associations between the posted items and their related activities. Each picture or icon can be displayed on a small laminated card and affixed to a Velcro strip in the proper sequence. Once created, students are taught to go to the schedule, check the picture representing the next activity, and then go to the indicated activity. When the activity is completed, the students return to the schedule, remove the icon, and place it in a "completed" section (e.g., another Velcro strip, a laminated pocket, etc.), and this process is continued throughout the day. Typically, visual schedules are individualized for each student's particular schedule as each learns the schedule following procedure.

Evaluating Class-Wide Behavior Supports. One of the ways that a PtP coach can support a teacher with these class-wide practices is to make use of a self-assessment tool to evaluate the classroom management practices currently in place in the teacher's classroom. In this scenario, the coach could provide a checklist to the teacher, prompting him or her to complete the checklist and then arrange a time to debrief following completion. This can then set the occasion for the identification of areas for improvement and a subsequent action plan developed for achieving targeted outcomes. The Classroom Management Self-Assessment Tool developed by Simonsen and colleagues (Simonsen, Fairbanks, Briesch, & Sugai, 2006) is an excellent example of a tool that can be used by coaches and teachers for this purpose. Another option is for the PtP coach to conduct a brief observation of the class, utilizing a classroom-management checklist, like the one shown in Table 11–8 to evaluate the extent to which effective class-wide behavior support strategies are being implemented. Similar to the use of a self-assessment, this observation would be followed by a meeting with the teacher to identify areas of strength and areas for growth noted by the coach on the checklist. The areas for growth could then also be targeted for improvement, and an action plan developed outlining what will be done and by what time so that follow-up observations or meetings can determine the outcome of these efforts.

Targeted Behavior Supports for Students With ASD: Addressed With Consultative Coaching

Even though the universal strategies described above provide a solid foundation for preventing and reducing many of the challenging behaviors that could otherwise interfere with the success of students with ASD, some students will need additional targeted behavior supports in order to be successful. Likewise, with an increased level of intensity with targeted supports, teachers may benefit from consultative coaching supporting their development and implementation of these support strategies. One example of a more intensive, evidence-based targeted behavior support is teaching self-management skills to students with ASD (National Autism Center, 2015). Self-management has been shown to be effective for high-functioning students with ASD (Wilkinson, 2008), students with limited expressive language (Pierce & Schreibman, 1994), students participating in general education settings (Koegel, Harrower, & Koegel, 1999), and has been demonstrated to improve a wide range of meaningful outcomes, including restricted and repetitive behaviors (Koegel & Koegel, 1990), as well as increased participation in social activities (Koegel, Koegel, Hurley, & Frea, 1992; Koegel & Frea, 1993).

There are five key steps to follow in setting up a self-management plan for students with ASD (Table 11–9). Thus, coaches should plan on providing ongoing support and follow-up to the teacher when implementing this approach, especially for the first time.

First, the coach and teacher must identify the behaviors to target for increase and/or decrease. Some examples of areas that could be targeted for increase include improved participation in classroom activities (e.g., academic engagement), social communicative skills

Table 11–8. Classroom Management Checklist

Observer	
Date	
School	
Classroom/ Teacher	
Comments	
Instructions	Using a scale from 1 to 5 (5 = Completely Agree, 3 = Somewhat Agree, 1 = Disagree), rank the extent to which you agree with each statement regarding the current status of, or current practice in the focus classroom.

Classroom Management Feature		Pre	Post	Follow-up
1.	Are rules, routines, and procedures posted in a manner that is easy to see?			
2.	Are rules, routines, and procedures posted in a manner that all can read or understand (visuals)?			
3.	Are classroom rules positively stated with no more than five identified?			
4.	Are the rules worded in observable and measurable terms?			
5.	Are the rules posted on a chart that is large enough for all to see?			
6.	Are the rules written in words that all can read and /or illustrated with graphics or icons?			
7.	Is the daily schedule of activities posted and reviewed regularly?			
8.	Are procedures for transitions and other relevant activities posted and regularly reviewed?			
9.	Are procedures taught in the settings and situations in which they are naturally needed?			
10.	Is there a method for posting changes to the schedule?			
11.	Are timelines adequate for the tasks planned?			

Table 11–8. *continued*

Classroom Management Feature		Pre	Post	Follow-up
12.	Does each student spend most of his or her time engaged in active learning activities, with little or no unstructured downtime?			
13.	Are classroom assistants actively involved with students in a manner that promotes their independence, learning, and interaction with peers?			
14.	Are the criteria used for earning reinforcers identified?			
15.	Is behavior-specific praise paired with the delivery of reinforcement?			
16.	Is behavior-specific praise (or other reinforcement) provided at a rate of five positives to every one corrective statement?			
17.	Are reinforcers (verbal, nonverbal, items, activities) available to all who earn them?			
18.	Are reinforcers varied and individualized?			
19.	Are error correction strategies delivered in a calm, positive manner prior to escalation of behavior?			
20.	Are error-correction strategies delivered consistently and in a timely manner?			

Table 11–9. Steps for Setting Up a Self-Management Plan

1. Identify Target Behavior(s)
2. Select an Array of Reinforcing Strategies
3. Choose a Recording Strategy
4. Teach Student to Identify/Record Target Behavior(s)
5. Fade Self-Management Components to Build Independence

(e.g. appropriate greetings), appropriate behaviors that are incompatible with, and/or preferable to identified challenging behavior (e.g., teaching hands in pockets while walking to replace stereotypical hand waving), and so on. Examples of behaviors targeted for decrease could include any identified challenging behavior, such as stereotypy, aggression, inappropriate vocalizations, and so on. The key to this first step is to operationally define the targeted behavior(s) using observable and measurable terms, as these will later need to be recorded. The second step is to select an array of reinforcement strategies to strengthen the new behaviors to be self-managed, or to reinforce the absence of challenging behaviors. These should include strategies for immediate reinforcement following target behaviors and student recording, as well as backup reinforcement options when longer-term goals are met. As mentioned in the classroom management section previously, conducting brief preference assessments with the student just prior to the start of each self-management period can increase the likelihood that the selected item or event will serve to reinforce the targeted behavior. After selecting reinforcers, the third step is for coaches and teachers to identify the way in which the targeted behavior will be recorded. This step includes deciding between a frequency count method or an interval recording method. (See Chapter 8 for a more detailed description of these two data collection methods.) Depending on which method is selected, there will be a corresponding strategy that will need to be used to allow the student to self-record his or her behavior. For a frequency count, the student will need a way to count the number of times he or she displays the targeted behavior. For a behavior expected to be displayed at a low frequency, a simple teacher-made paper and pencil form can be used allowing the student to self-record his or her behavior. However, for high-frequency behaviors or those that need to be used in a variety of settings (e.g.,

social communicative skills), the student may need a portable device to discretely monitor use of the targeted behaviors (e.g., golf counters). When an interval recording method is selected, typically to track the absence of a challenging behavior, the student will need a cue at the end of the interval to prompt him or her to record the performance (e.g., a prerecorded tone) on the self-recording sheet. In this case, for longer time intervals or when the student is self-recording in multiple settings, the device used to prompt recording will also need to be portable and discrete (e.g., a programmed, repeating, and tactile alarm on a cell phone or other device). Fourth, the student will need to be taught to discriminate between the desired and undesired behaviors so that he or she can identify when the targeted performance criteria have been met. When teaching discrimination initially, teachers should focus reinforcement on accurate identification, rather than actual performance or the behavior. Then, once student recording consistently matches teacher recording, reinforcement can be shifted to be contingent on performance. Periodic comparisons between student and teacher recordings may need to be conducted over time, or in new settings, to ensure the accuracy of independent student self-recording. However, over time students with ASD can become quite independent with monitoring and recording their own behavior. The final step in the self-management process is to gradually fade out elements of the intervention in order to increase independent self-management skills on the part of the student. This fading process should be done systematically, and typically begins with the fading of any adult-delivered prompts. After the removal of adult prompts, the performance criteria for earning reinforcement can be gradually increased (increase length of recording intervals, or number of instances behavior is to be performed). Next, the schedule of reinforcement can be thinned by increasing the number of successful intervals required of the student before access to reinforcement is provided. Finally, the physical proximity of adults can be decreased allowing the student to engage in independent self-management.

Consultative coaching would be helpful to teachers when implementing self-management strategies, in that this level of coaching provides for follow-along support from a more experienced mentor. As self-management approaches should be modified for each participating student, and entail multiple steps in planning and implementation, ongoing coaching can increase the likelihood that self-management skills will be taught effectively. An excellent resource for coaches and teachers for planning and implementing self-management strategies is the Self-Management Manual available from the Koegel Autism Center at the University of California, Santa Barbara (Koegel, Koegel, & Parks, 1992). This manual allows coaches and teachers to walk through the steps for setting up a self-management strategy for a given student, resulting in a fully developed self-management approach designed to address that student's specific needs.

Individualized Behavior Supports for Students With ASD: Addressed With Intensive Coaching

Teacher preparation programs around the country vary greatly to the extent with which they effectively prepare educators of students with ASD (Scheuermann, Webber, Boutot, & Goodwin, 2003). As a result, at the individualized level of behavior support, teachers may themselves seek a more intensive level of coaching support to effectively provide intensive behavior supports to students with severe challenging behavior. Additionally, when it is determined that a student is in need of intensive, individualized behavior supports, it is critical that a broader team convene to oversee this process. The issues presented in Chapter 6 about working with a team are critical at this stage. Coaches may need to support teachers to engage in activities spanning those covered in Sections II and III of this book when providing intensive, individualized behavior supports. The specific details required in developing comprehensive, individualized behavior intervention plans for students with ASD are beyond the scope of this chapter, but the main features of this approach are summarized below. Coaches and teachers are encouraged to make use of the many available resources on designing behavior intervention plans, some of which are identified in Table 11–10.

The first step in designing this level of behavior support is to engage in a collaborative process of identifying the

Table 11–10. Resources for Developing and Implementing Comprehensive Positive Behavior Support Plans

Resources	Location
IRIS Star Legacy Module: Functional Behavioral Assessment: Identifying the Reasons for Problem Behavior and Developing a Behavior Plan	Available from the IRIS Center: http://iris.peabody.vanderbilt.edu/
Facilitator's Guide: Positive Behavioral Support	Available from the Florida Positive Behavior Support Project: http://flpbs.fmhi.usf.edu/
BIP Desk Reference Manual	Available from the PENT: Positive Environments, Network of Trainers: http://www.pent.ca.gov/

goals and anticipated outcomes of the behavior support plan. Many teams have utilized Person-Centered Planning approaches to facilitate the goal identification process (Kincaid & Fox, 2002). In person-centered planning, the team (described in Chapter 6) goes through a planning process, where they identify the strengths of the student, along with current areas of concern, and then develop an action plan to address the current concerns and to build upon student and family strengths. Teams often come away from this process feeling more aware of the student's needs and their own role in supporting the student. Person-centered planning has also been used when there are major barriers to effective collaboration among team members. Because it focuses on identifying positive outcomes that team members agree on, it can lead to improvements in team functioning for team members struggling to collaborate. Because this process focuses on student strengths (and functions as a strengths-based assessment), parents often report that the person-centered planning process was the first time their needs, perspectives, and concerns related to their child with ASD had been heard and acknowledged.

Ultimately, the following areas are recommended for goal identification: (a) define specific challenging behaviors to decrease; (b) define specific appropriate behaviors to increase; (c) pinpoint circumstances in which intervention will occur (i.e., when, where, with whom, etc.); and (d) identify lifestyle changes desired (e.g., participation in integrated activities, enhanced independence and satisfaction, expanded social networks, etc.).

The next step in designing intensive behavior supports is to operationally define the behavior targeted for increase and decrease. As covered in Chapter 8, and in the section above on Self-Management, an operational definition of behavior is one that is observable and measurable. A few suggestions to keep in mind when describing behavior operationally include using exact quotes of what the student said, describing the sequence of events in the exact order in which they occurred, describing what did/did not happen, and describing body language.

A major feature of effective behavior supports is the use of a Functional Behavior Assessment (FBA) as the basis for plan development. In conducting an FBA, information on antecedents, or events and conditions that precede/trigger the target behavior and consequences, or events and conditions that follow/reinforce the target behavior will need to be gathered. This information is then summarized in a hypothesis statement, in order to clarify the function, or purpose, of the targeted challenging behavior(s). Possible functions of behavior generally fall into two major categories: (a) positive reinforcement, or what the student gains access to as a result of the challenging behavior, or (b) negative reinforcement, or what the student avoids as a result of the challenging behavior. Within each of these two main categories, the function of a behavior can be further broken down into subcategories including attention (peer and/or adult), tangibles/activities, and automatic/sensory stimuli. For instance, a possible function of challenging behavior could be negative reinforcement exemplified by avoidance of social interactions with peers. Likewise, another example could be positive reinforcement exemplified by gaining access to a preferred activity (e.g., games on a tablet device). There are numerous examples of possible functions of behavior; however, it is critical to the develop-

ment of effective behavior supports that they be identified in the context of these two categories. Ensuring such alignment in the hypothesis statement of the FBA allows for the selection of appropriate and effective strategies for inclusion in the behavior plan.

Three elements of behavior support plans include (a) strategies designed to address identified antecedent conditions and triggers, referred to as *preventive, proactive*, or *antecedent-based strategies*; (b) strategies designed to teach functionally equivalent replacement behaviors, referred to as *instructional* or *educative strategies*; and (c) strategies designed to both reinforce appropriate behaviors and to withhold/limit access to reinforcement following challenging behaviors, referred to as *consequence* or *functional strategies*. Comprehensive, behavior support plans will consist of multiple intervention strategies all linked back to the particular function of the student's target behavior(s).

A key consideration for implementing the behavior support plan is to evaluate the fidelity, or accuracy, with which the behavior intervention strategies are actually implemented by those tasked with their implementation. Given that multiple strategies are typically implemented in a single student's behavior support plan, frequently by multiple adults, the coach and teacher will want to develop a plan for assessing the extent to which behavior plan components are being delivered. Often this can be achieved by asking each adult tasked with the responsibility of implementing a strategy to report data on their use of it coupled with regular check-ins with the teacher. During these check-ins, the teacher can review the data on implementation, gain an understanding of the other adult's sense for how intervention strategies are working, probe the adult's level of satisfaction with using the strategies, and action plan next steps regarding ongoing implementation and/or revision of the plan.

Last, the coach and teacher will need to ensure the development of progress monitoring strategies to evaluate the impact of the behavior plan on student behavior. Making use of the data collection methods and forms covered in Chapter 8 can provide for ongoing evaluation of the extent to which behavior plan components address the behavioral needs of the student. Data can also point to the possible need for revision of the behavior support plan, either to improve its effectiveness, or to initiate the gradual fading of supports to build student independence.

Summary

Coaches can support teachers via high-quality coaching providing the appropriate levels of intensity to support improvement in restricted, repetitive behaviors, interests, and activities of students with ASD, which can often interfere with social and academic success. Determining relative areas of teacher strength and need allows coaches to match an appropriate level of support utilizing a peer-to-peer, consultative, or intensive coaching model. Likewise, working with the teacher to identify varying levels of

student need relative to behavioral functioning, the coach provides a framework for developing appropriate, evidence-based behavior supports at universal, targeted, and/or individual levels for students with ASD.

End-of-Chapter Questions

1. Suppose you are a coach supporting a teacher in developing a lesson plan for teaching classroom rules. Using Table 11–4, identify an appropriate classroom rule and complete a sample lesson plan for the teacher to use to teach this rule.

2. Suppose you are a coach supporting a teacher in developing a lesson plan for teaching classroom procedures. Using Table 11–6, identify a classroom activity, and develop a sample lesson plan for the teacher to use to teach the associated procedures for this activity.

3. Following the guidelines outlined in Table 11–9 for developing a plan to teach self-management skills to students with ASD, design a self-management strategy for a student you work with. Be sure to develop detailed strategies for each of the five steps presented.

4. Students with ASD may display restrictive, repetitive behaviors, interests, and activities for a variety of reasons. Using the information provided in this chapter related to identifying the function of a behavior,

please provide two different possible Hypothesis Statements (*antecedents*, *behavior*, consequences, and *function*) for the following student target behavior: "Repetitive waving of hands in front of eyes."

5. For one of the Hypothesis Statements developed for question #4, please provide sample behavior support strategies appropriate for the scenario selected. Be sure to include at least one strategy from each of the behavior support plan categories identified in the text (i.e., *proactive/preventative, instructional/educative,* and *consequence/functional*).

References

Cohen, M. J., & Sloan, D. L. (2007). *Visual supports for people with autism: A guide for parents and professionals.* Bethesda, MD: Woodbine House.

Cooper, J., Heron, T., & Heward, W. (2007). *Applied behavior analysis* (2nd ed.). Upper Saddle River, NJ: Prentice-Hall.

Kincaid, D., & Fox, L. (2002). Person-centered planning and positive behavior support. In S. Holburn & P. Vietze (Eds.), *Research and practice in person-centered planning* (pp. 29–50). Baltimore, MD: Paul H. Brookes.

Koegel, L. K., Harrower, J. K., & Koegel, R. L. (1999). Support for children with developmental disabilities in full inclusion classrooms through self-management. *Journal of Positive Behavior Interventions, 1,* 26–34.

Koegel, L. K., Koegel, R. L., Hurley, C., & Frea, W. D. (1992). Improving social skills and disruptive behavior in children with autism through self-management. *Journal of Applied Behavior Analysis, 25,* 341–353.

Koegel, L. K., Koegel, R. L., & Parks, D. R. (1992). *How to teach self-management skills to people with severe disabilities: A training manual.* Santa Barbara, CA: University of California.

Koegel, R. L., & Frea, W. D. (1993). Treatment of social behavior in autism through the modification of pivotal social skills. *Journal of Applied Behavior Analysis, 26,* 369–377.

Koegel, R. L., & Koegel, L. K. (1990). Extended reductions in stereotypic behavior of students with autism through a self-management treatment package. *Journal of Applied Behavior Analysis, 23,* 119–127.

National Autism Center. (2015). *Findings and conclusions: National standards project, phase 2.* Randolph, MA: Author.

Pas, E. T., Bradshaw, C. P., Hershfeldt, P. A., & Leaf, P. J. (2010). A multilevel exploration of the influence of teacher efficacy and burnout on response to student problem behavior and school-based service use. *School Psychology Quarterly, 25*(1), 13–27.

Pierce, K. L. & Schreibman, L. (1994). Teaching daily living skills to children with autism in unsupervised settings through pictorial self-management. *Journal of Applied Behavior Analysis, 27*(3), 471–481.

Scheuermann, S., Webber, J., Boutot, E. A., & Goodwin, M. (2003). Problems with personnel preparation in autism spectrum disorders. *Focus on Autism and Other Developmental Disabilities, 18*(3), 197–206.

Simonsen, B., Fairbanks, S., Briesch, A., Myers, D., & Sugai, G. (2008). Evidence-based practices in classroom management: Considerations for research to practice. *Education and Treatment of Children, 31*(3), 351–380.

Simonsen, B., Fairbanks, S., Briesch, A., & Sugai, G. (2006). *Classroom management: Self-assessment revised.* Storrs, CT: Center on Positive Behavioral Interventions and Supports, University of Connecticut.

Sugai, G., Horner, R. H., Dunlap, G., Hieneman, M., Lewis, T. J., Nelson, C. M., . . . Ruef, M. (2000). Applying positive behavior support and functional behavioral assessment in schools. *Journal of Positive Behavior Interventions, 2*(3), 131–143.

Tobin, T., Horner, R., Vincent, C., & Swain-Bradway, J. (2012). If discipline referral rates for the school as a whole are reduced, will rates for students with disabilities also be reduced? *OSEP Technical Assistance Center on PBIS: Evaluation Briefs, Issue 12.*

Wilkinson, L. A. (2008). Self-management for children with high-functioning autism spectrum disorders. *Intervention in School and Clinic, 43*(3), 150–157.

Wong, C., Odom, S. L., Hume, K. Cox, A. W., Fettig, A., Kucharczyk, S., . . . Schultz, T. R. (2014). *Evidence-based practices for children, youth, and young adults with Autism Spectrum Disorder.* Chapel Hill, NC: University of North Carolina, Frank Porter Graham Child Development Institute, Autism Evidence-Based Practice Review Group.

CHAPTER 12

Transition Planning and Coaching: Using a Life Course Outcome Mapping Approach

What the best and wisest parent wants for his own child,
that must the community want for all its children.

—John Dewey

Chapter Objectives

- Introduce and discuss the value of transition planning for students with autism spectrum disorder (ASD) from school entry through school exit.

- Describe Life Course Outcome Mapping (LCOM) and Life Course Individualized Education Program (IEP) planning for students with ASD, and their educational teams, including parents and caregivers.

- Identify how three levels of coaching support can assist in transition planning throughout schooling.

The vignette in Box 12–1 is telling. The mother unknowingly asked realistic questions about transition to adulthood prior to her son having a diagnosis. Who would have guessed some 30 years ago that transition services for students with disabilities in general, and students with autism in particular, would become an essential component of educational and adulthood planning?

According to IDEA 2004, transition planning starts at age 16, so that students along with caregivers can begin to fashion a reasonable plan for transitioning from the safety of the daily classroom routine to the world of employment, postsecondary schooling, community engagement, and independent living. IDEA defines transition services as a coordinated set of activities for a child with a disability that is

- designed to be within a results-oriented process, and focused on improving the academic and functional achievement of the individual with a disability to facilitate the individual's movement from school to postschool activities including postsecondary education, vocational education, integrated employment (including supported employment), continuing and

---

Box 12–1. Vignette: A Mother's Cry for Help

Years ago a friend came banging on my door screaming at the top of her lungs that her child had autism. She had come back from the doctor's office and he had handed her a magazine article on autism telling her to take it home and read it because her son might have some of those characteristics. Crying, she asked, "Is it true? Does Andy have autism? What does it mean? Will he ever have a job? Will he ever get married? Where will he live? Will he have friends? Tell me if he has autism? How will he take care of himself, and how will we take care of him?" I remember this interaction as if it were yesterday. This mom's pleas were appeals that I had heard before as a special educator. I comforted her, telling her I was here for her to talk with about Andy's future; just give me a call or knock on the door. I also gave her resources and the name of a professional that she could talk with about her son, encouraging her to make contact as soon as possible. She left still crying, partly because of the insensitivity of the doctor, but mostly because of the unknown future: a fear of the uncertainty of her son's adult life, that she voiced with her initial questions when she burst through my door.

adult education, adult services, independent living, or community participation;

■ based on the individual's needs, taking into account the individual's strengths, preferences, and interests, and includes instruction, related services, community experiences, the development of employment and other postschool adult living objectives and, when appropriate, acquisition of daily living skills and a functional vocational evaluation. [34 CFR 300.43 (a)] [20 U.S.C. 1401(34)] (Building the Legacy of IDEA 2004, IDEA Regulations, Secondary Transition).

Federal law stipulates what should occur when students turn 16 in regard to preparing them for school-to-work transitions. Educational research identifies vital information about the long-term benefits of this process. For example, Taylor and colleagues (Taylor & Seltzer, 2012; Taylor, Smith, & Mailick, 2014) clearly point out that a supported work environment for individuals with ASD increases socially appropriate behavior, quality of life, and cognitive abilities (Taylor & Seltzer 2012; Taylor et al., 2014). Nevertheless, according to Friedman, Warfield, and Parish (2013), overall transition outcomes for individuals with ASD reflect uneven attainment of skills, resulting in poor secondary and postsecondary education outcomes with very few individuals who ultimately participate in employment as adults. Despite the positive impact of adult employment,

families are left with fragmented systems of care once their youth with ASD transition out of entitled IDEA services for children and into adulthood (Friedman et al., 2013). Friedman et al. suspect that current models of school-based transition planning are inadequate given such poor outcomes in vocational training and employment for adults with ASD. Additionally, there is a shortage of appropriate opportunities for independence, and concurrently a long wait list for adult services (Gerhardt & Lainer, 2011; Howlin, Goode, Hutton, & Rutter, 2005).

Taylor and Seltzer (2010) examined the changes in behavioral phenotype (symptoms) in individuals with ASD before and after they exit the public school system and enter adulthood. Results showed that on average, symptomology-associated ASD that includes repetitive behaviors, stereotyped interests, impairments in social reciprocity, and impairments in verbal communication all improved prior to exiting high school, including a reduction in maladaptive behaviors (behaviors that include aggression, self-injury, and noncompliance). However, once these individuals exited high school, the improvements in these symptoms significantly slowed down. According to the study, the "turning point" of transitioning out of high school has a disruptive effect in behavioral phenotype in individuals with ASD, with significant slowing of improvement in most symptom areas and cognitive development (Taylor & Seltzer, 2010).

Taylor and Seltzer (2010) believe this pattern of slowed improvement is reflective of less stimulating adult occupational and day activities compared to what students experienced in high school. They found that 74% of young adults with ASD and comorbid intellectual disability (ID) were receiving adult day services, while 25% of young adults with ASD and without ID did not have occupational, educational, or day activities. These findings have significant implications for stimulating job opportunities and effective adult services for youth with ASD. Unfortunately, according to Gerhardt and Lainer (2011), the vast majority of adults with ASD in their study (90%) were either unemployed or underemployed, and many went without appropriate services.

Billstedt, Gillberg, and Gillberg (2005) conducted a follow-up study of 120 individuals with ASD from childhood to adulthood. They found that 57% of the sample of individuals had *very poor outcomes* (i.e., were unable to have any kind of independent existence, and were without any verbal or nonverbal communication); 21% had *poor outcomes* (i.e., no independent social progress with some verbal or nonverbal communication); 13% had *restricted but acceptable outcomes* (i.e., they had the same characteristics of the poor outcome group but were accepted by peers); 8% had *fair outcomes* (i.e., being employed or living independently with two or more friends), and none had *good outcomes* (i.e., being employed and living independently).

Migliore, Butterworth, and Zalewska (2014) investigated the trend in youth with ASD and the types of services associated with vocational rehabilitation (VR) and employment outcomes from the services accessed, compared with

youth with other disabilities. In order to achieve economic self-sufficiency, employment programs have been emphasized across many states, and many have adopted "employment first" policies that receive funding priority. Combining the employment first policies with the population increase in youth with ASD translates to a substantial increase of employment services needed by those advancing into adulthood. Additionally, results showed the number of youth with ASD exiting vocational rehabilitation (VR) programs doubled in recent years, yet remained relatively small compared with other disability groups. Only about half the youth who received VR services exited the program with integrated employment, and the number who received VR services declined slightly over time. Consequently, receiving VR services is indicative of progress toward employment (Migliore et al., 2014). Considering these current trends for those with ASD, it is essential to further investigate the benefits associated with vocational training and supported employment and fund these kinds of opportunities (Garcia, 2015).

The research and statistics on post-educational outcomes for individuals with ASD sounds a dire alarm. How do we begin to address transition in a clear and cogent fashion and prior to a student turning 16 years of age? How do educators, parents, and coaches begin to think of transition earlier, possibly as early as a child's initial diagnosis? A viable and needed approach to offset the trend of poor transition planning to adulthood would be to develop an outcomes-based service delivery model wherein educators plan prospectively. Planning prospectively and designing educational experiences with the ultimate goal of independent living, gainful employment, and other postsecondary living objectives then becomes the lens that educators, families, and coaches look through. This is of utmost importance because the future for individuals with ASD and their families is always just around the corner. Keeping the first vignette of this chapter in mind helps us realize that parents anticipate the future almost immediately when problems are suspected in early childhood. They look to the medical and educational community to provide services with the hope that someday their child will be independent, have friends, hold down a job, and enjoy an enviable life (Turnbull, 2010).

Traditional Transition Planning

At the age of 16, the IEP team develops a comprehensive transition plan including interagency responsibilities and other needed ancillary services. Unless they graduate with a high school diploma in hand, students with special needs are entitled to the right to attend school until the age of 22. However, rights must be transferred over to the student when they turn 18 years of age. As stated in the federal law, transition services must be in concert with the student's interests and preferences that could include employment or varied community experiences, postsecondary goals, employ-

ability skill training, daily living assistance, and a vocational evaluation. When students are involved in the IEP process and are given an opportunity to develop their own goals about their aspirations, it gives them control over the outcome of the plan as they work with the educational team. Conversely, if the student is unable to participate in the IEP transition process, then parents or caregivers can shape a plan that makes sense. Related services such as transportation, rehabilitation counseling, and social work services to help students succeed in the transition from school to work also may be necessary. Transition services are usually provided by someone knowledgeable about the process with the requisite training to ensure that the skills and knowledge needed by the student are consistent with the student's goals and aims. Vocational trainers, job coaches, job training coordinators, career specialists, and other related transition service personnel provide support in this planning process.

Nontraditional Transition Planning: Life Course Outcome Mapping

What is needed is a radical shift of focus in typical posteducational planning. What if transition training started as the child enters school? What if, as articulated by Wehman (2013), all special education personnel implement progressive, or outcome oriented, planning to begin to move the student in the direction of a meaningful life experience with early discussion about employment, leisure, community involvement, education, and independent living? A review of this topic by Stewart and colleagues (2010), who analyzed over 500 articles on transition services for students across the spectrum of disabilities, reported that services, though improving, have not rendered the results hoped for or mandated by U.S. law. King et al. (2005) argue that a holistic, lifelong view of transition is imperative so that as Stewart, Law, Rosenbaum, and Williams (2001) indicate, youth and parents do not feel like "they have been dropped off a cliff" once they reach adulthood.

The feeling of being suddenly dropped from a supportive educational environment to a landscape of unknowns highlights the importance of having students participate in normalized environments as soon as they are capable. Although the severity of symptoms ranges from severe to mild on the autism spectrum, preparation for transition from one learning environment to another needs to begin as soon as a child with ASD enters school, even before, and should be reinforced consistently at home. If not, individuals with this disability will continue to be cared for by their families until they can no longer provide the necessary support needed. The vignette in Box 12–2 emphasizes this point.

The young man in this vignette, who was verbal and most capable, could have completed the entire purchase routine himself. It might have taken a few more minutes, but assuredly, this would be a more desirable outcome. This young man with ASD is potentially a good candidate for the proposed concept

and transition planning process of *life course outcome mapping* (Figure 12–1). Life course outcome transition planning starts upon school entry and continues throughout formal schooling, ensuring that students with ASD have the requisite training and opportunities to promote self-determination for life after special education. For this very capable young man, waiting for cues and prompts from his mother indicates that he may not have been given the necessary tools and practice to become independent, which we see his former teacher reflect upon.

To offset the sense of helplessness individuals with an ASD and their families often feel after formal schooling ends, the remainder of this chapter comprehensively explores the concept of LCOM. A sample of how a peer-to-peer coach or teacher might implement a *life course IEP* appears in the life course outcome map for an elementary student, James. A key component of this process, thoughtful prospective planning, shows the viability of the approach. Along with the LCOM developed by a peer-to-peer coach, consultative and intensive coaching delivery models (see Chapter 5) can also be implemented to assist educators in implementing this type of forward transition planning.

Initial Life Course Outcome Planning at School Entry

At the first IEP meeting, when a student enters school, the educational team can ask parents or caregivers to entertain the notion of thinking about their child's future, discussing a process for beginning to determine outcomes after their

---

Box 12–2. Vignette: Coffee Shop Follow-Up

I couldn't help noticing a person behind me in line at the coffee shop talking. I glanced back and a former student of mine, now in his early 20s, was talking with his mother about his order. They didn't see me, so I took the opportunity to observe how well he would do making his order. Having developed a transition plan for him when he was in my class, I was really interested in how he was doing now. What caught my attention was his repetitive conversation about his ensuing order of "pumpkin cake, pumpkin cake, pumpkin cake, hot chocolate with whipped cream." He was next in line after me, and when he finally arrived to place his order, he quickly moved over to the display case to make sure the pumpkin cake was available. After scanning, and noticing it was there he ordered, "pumpkin cake, pumpkin cake and hot chocolate with whipped cream." He was most anxious and thrown off when the cashier asked if he wanted the pumpkin cake heated. His reply was, "pumpkin cake, pumpkin cake," quickly followed by his mother interceding for him letting the cashier know that cold was fine. He then fumbled with his money to pay for the purchase, giving the cashier much more than was due (and not using the "dollar-up" method). He stood very anxiously moving his head from side to side and then rocking back and forth waiting for the cashier to hand him back his change. His mother instructed him to put a tip in the tip jar, which he did. He moved over to the order pickup area and commenced rocking. All in all, considering the intensity of the loud stimuli at the coffee shop, he did fairly well handling himself with help from his mother. When I greeted him and his mother, they both seemed happy to see me, and I got the sense that they both wished he could still be receiving the special education services provided while he was still in school. Despite his mother's kind words, I left the impromptu follow-up observation feeling like more could have been done to prepare him for life after school.

---

child leaves formal schooling between 18 and 22 years of age. Understandably, there may be some trepidation, but if posed as an opportunity to discuss what parents would ultimately like their child to achieve in school to prepare their child for postschool success, it begins a practical dialogue, and most likely the

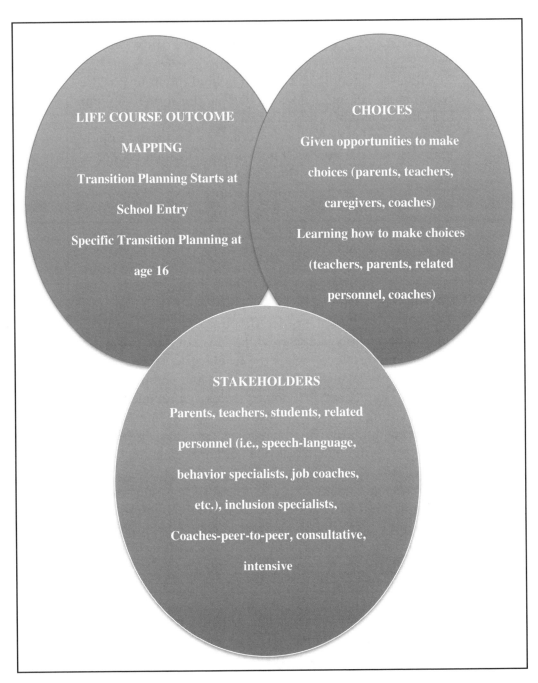

Figure 12–1. Conceptual frame for life course outcome mapping.

response will be positive. The teacher can share the concept of LCOM as the process the team will use to stimulate conversation about the family's hopes and dreams for their child, much as is done in the person-centered planning approach (Clark, Knab, & Kincaid, 2005).

At the LCOM meeting, the teacher asks the first pertinent and far-reaching question, "What are your hopes and dreams for your son when he leaves high school?" It is all but guaranteed that parents would not say "to become proficient in Biology." They most likely would say that they want their son to have a good life and be as independent as possible. They might even talk about employment options that they think would be beneficial for him. No different than parents with typically developing children, they also might discuss marriage and children.

At this first meeting, the outcomes are discussed and written down as long-term future goals. The next question is, "How best can we help your child attain the life course you have outlined?" Most likely, the response would be similar, once again, to parents of typically developing children at the school: make sure he or she interacts with peers, learns the social skills necessary for interacting with others, and gains skills to reach the long-term goals and dreams we have for him or her. To realize these eventual goals, students with ASD need to be given every opportunity to make choices in the most natural and engaging manner possible. Limiting choice-making mitigates against reaching long-range goals, and hopes and dreams parents may have for their children (as suggested earlier in the vignette in Box 12–2). Involving as many stakeholders as possible provides the foundation for transition planning when using the LCOM process (see the "Stakeholders" Circle in Figure 12–1). All stakeholders then become responsible for ensuring that students from school entry to school exit have multiple oppor-

tunities to make decisions and choices that could allow them to live independently with marketable skills (see the "Choices" Circle in Figure 12–1).

The realization that transition needs to begin as early as a student enters school can be somewhat daunting for teachers, parents, and coaches. How does one keep that long-range goal in mind while still dealing with day-to-day training and skill development, which might be incremental at best for many students with ASD? First, the teacher, who as stipulated throughout this book also wears the hat of a peer-to-peer coach, now incorporates future goals as a context for implementing short-term and annual goals. The LCOM process provides a salient vehicle for a parent and/or coach to endorse team transition goals and the means to implementing those goals.

For transition planning to begin when a student with ASD first enters school requires a shift in thinking. In all likelihood, thinking about the future for a 3-year-old entering school for the first time presents challenges for school personnel as well as for parents or caregivers. Parents are just getting their first taste of schooling and what it portends for their child. Having to think about something so far in the future is daunting and anxiety producing. Therefore, mapping a postschool outcome in a clear, stepwise fashion can help relieve tension giving stakeholders a roadmap to follow. The LCOM Form (Table 12–1) and steps outlined in the next section provide a viable way to identify needs and make instructional decisions that will potentially prepare students for postschool opportunities.

Table 12–1. Life Course Outcome Mapping for Postschool Transition Form

Student's Name	Parents' Names	Grade Level	Date

Life Course Vision (hopes and dreams after 22 years of age)

Who will partner with making the vision a reality?   When (school year/semester)?

Life Course IEP Present Levels of Performance   What's working to realize the dream for the future?   Obstacles in realizing the dream and future aspirations

What are our goals? Keep expectations realistic. Progress from more general statements when students are young to more specific statements in middle and high school. Goal 1: Goal 2: Goal 3:

Table 12–1. *continued*

How do we plan to meet the goals?
Benchmarks
Activities

Life Course Outcome Map

1. Create the vision with all stakeholders. What are your hopes and dreams for your child when he or she graduates at 22 years of age? Do you hope he or she develops interests to occupy his or her time, find and develop a talent such as music, art, a sport, be prepared to work hard, know the difference between right and wrong, develop friendships, find a lifetime mate or partner, live independently or semi-independently, have enough money to pay bills, establish a career or hold down a job, and participate in the community in which he or she belongs?

2. Identify all the individuals or groups (i.e., teachers, instructional assistants, related service providers, behavior technicians, and other IEP team members) that will influence the process from beginning until the end of schooling years.

3. Develop a *life course IEP*. The goals should be directly related to the vision and should (a) include present levels of performance related to the vision. Identify any obstacles, and also determine what's working and what is not working for a given student. (b) Identify the goals and timelines. Be realistic and clearly delineate expectations. And, (c) specify benchmarks and activities for improvement and how you plan to reach life course goals.

4. Decide on how the team will organize themselves to make sure the vision is operationalized. For example, if the student has an assigned behavior or support specialist, then in the early grade years there might be more direct assistance with less direct support as the student moves into upper elementary grades. At the middle and high school level, the student makes his or her own decisions and choices as much as possible,

and the adult specialist provides less direct contact and support.

5. Keep an *outcome journal* to collect data about the progress related to the life course IEP over time as well as general comments related to overall social engagement essential for success in life after special education concludes. The outcome journal could be notes logged in a computer file, iPhone, iPad, or spiral bound notebook with dates. The entries could be simple bullet points or in narrative format. Journal notes should be shared with staff members. The outcome journal information would be sent as an attachment in some electronic format that is accessible to all stakeholders; if handwritten, they are included in the student's cumulative folder.

Caveat: Because a life course IEP is not mandated by law, parents would need to request that LCOM documents (life course IEP and outcome journal) be included as part of the documentation to be forwarded to the next teacher or school. The LCOM process should be shared with the student's next teacher as well as any discussion about the journaling process. Parents familiar with the LCOM concept will most likely catalyze this type of transition planning from an early age throughout the child's academic career until a school district, inclusion coaches, and teachers unfamiliar with it embrace the concept.

As mentioned previously, transition to adult life starts as soon as the child enters school. Educators who part-

ner with parents to help their children realize postschool goals send a clear message that the skills learned will be essential for independent living. Developing a life course IEP helps crystallize the fact that specific goals directed to helping the family and student realize basic opportunities afforded to typically developing students can also be fulfilled by individuals with ASD. Charting that course as the child progresses through school with key stakeholders along the way increases the likelihood that a student will leave formal schooling with skills that allow for meaningful participation in postschool activities.

Peer-to-Peer Coaching and Life Course Outcome Mapping

Most direct services for students with ASD occur at the classroom level with a certificated teacher in charge. Oftentimes the teacher then assumes the role of a peer coach, helping instructional assistants, behavior specialists, volunteers, and parents understand the significance and meaning of varied instructional approaches utilized in the classroom. With so many day-to-day instructional and managerial responsibilities, developing a LCOM along with a life course IEP may feel like a burden to a teacher. On the other hand, thinking about the future with a team of professionals, including the family, could be exhilarating. A conversation about hopes and dreams alters the way professionals think about teaching students. Further, if the teacher has the opportunity for peer-to-peer coaching with staff members and parents via LCOM, he or she might incorporate different service delivery and instructional options, setting up forward thinking with her team. Imagine the following scenario.

James is an 11-year-old student in Mrs. Clay's class. He communicates his needs with basic sentence structure and gets along with his peers and teachers. In fact, he takes on leadership roles in the classroom as line manager and peer helper. His social skills are quite good within the classroom; however, on the playground and other unstructured settings, his repetitive behavior of rocking is noticeable. Reducing rocking behavior is one of his IEP goals. At an open house for the school, the parents seemingly out of the blue, asked Mrs. Clay about James's future. They asked her, "Where does she see James in 10 years and beyond?" They followed up with questions about whether she thought he could live independently; will he have typical friends; will he live in a group home and maybe hold down a job? Mrs. Clay was most empathetic with the parents' queries, indicating that because James was only 11 years old and in elementary school, she was focused on the IEP goals at hand, and had not really given much thought to postschool transition. She asked the parents if they could identify one or two of the long-range goals that were most important to them. They responded by saying that they would like James to hold down a job where he could work

with people, for example, at a grocery store, hardware store, or department store. They believed that James could learn rudimentary tasks associated with stocking shelves, bagging groceries, and working in a stockroom. They also wanted him to live independently learning to ride the bus back and forth to work and share an apartment with others who would understand him and be friendly toward him. Mrs. Clay wrote down the parents wish/dream list, and said she would look for a way to implement this above and beyond James's current IEP goals. She would also communicate the list to her staff, so once she figured out the best course of action, she could begin to coach them on how to focus on postschool transition, an area she was sure the school team had not fully considered.

Although Mrs. Clay did not have resources readily at hand, the LCOM process would seem like a good match to the family's hopes and desires. Table 12–2 illustrates what it might look like for James and his parents, spelling out how the teacher would coach her team working toward those goals.

For this example, the teacher/peer-to-peer (PtP) coach would review the life course map with educational staff members pointing out all aspects of the map and asking for input. After discussion, the PtP coach would problem solve with the team how to implement the life course map and conduct a weekly or bimonthly meeting with staff members to talk about life course goals and adjust benchmarks or activities. At the weekly or bimonthly meeting, the PtP coach shares the outcome

Table 12–2. James's Life Course Outcome Map

Life Course Outcome Mapping for Postschool Transition			
Student's Name	Parents' Names	Grade Level and Name of Teacher	Date
James Olsen	Marie and Brad Olsen	5th, Mrs. Clay	September 2015

Life Course Vision (hopes and dreams after 22 years of age)

The family would like James to live independently and hold down a job that allows him to interact with people on a daily basis. He is social, and parents are certain that as an adult, James will thrive on adult interaction. He could work with people, at a grocery store, hardware store, or department store. The family believes that James could learn rudimentary tasks associated with stocking shelves, bagging groceries, or working in a stockroom. They would like him to ride the public bus back and forth to work and live with friends or individuals who understand him and are friendly toward him. They also feel that his schooling from this point forward should be aimed toward postschool life choices.

Who will partner in making the vision become a reality?

Mr. and Mrs. Olsen, grandfather, an older cousin who wants to become a special education teacher, classroom teacher, instructional assistants, school psychologist, speech-language pathologist, and other service providers.

When (school year/semester)?

Beginning in the Fall 2015 semester with quarterly check-ins to discuss James' progress as well as continuing the conversation about aspirations, hopes, and dreams for James.

Life Course IEP Present Levels of Performance

James is social and enjoys interacting with peers and adults. He likes watching TV, especially action movies and cartoons. He follows directions well, although at this age often needs reminders for step completion. He has assumed a few leadership positions in class and responds to praise and encouragement. Sometimes his repetitive behavior of rocking calls attention to itself; when he rocks he tends to "space out," not make eye contact, and retreat into his own world. However, with prompts and other learning supports he is able to cycle out of it fairly quickly. His communication is improving from simple to more complex sentence structure. His SLP continues to work with him in class on using his words to communicate requests and making comments, and has helped the teachers and instructional assistants know how to model communication. James also makes choices about food, clothes, and iPad games. All of these are skill areas that need to be reinforced regularly for James to be successful in postschool environments.

What's working to realize the dream for the future?

Choice making on a daily basis, offering more and different choices and reinforcing this behavior at school and home.

- Socially able to interact appropriately with peers and adults
- Follows directions
- Beginning to communicate with more complex sentences

Table 12–2. *continued*

Obstacles in realizing the dream and future aspirations

- Repetitive rocking behavior and difficulty interacting with others
- Making sure that each teacher receives prior Life Course IEP and develops a new one each year
- Social communication skills do not progress, which could limit adult interaction at an employment site

---

What are our goals? Keep expectations realistic. Progress from more general statements when students are young to more specific statements in middle and high school.

Goal 1: James will learn about city bus transportation

Goal 2: James will begin to learn how to pay for a bus fare with money or learn how to use the "Go To Pass" card

Goal 3: James will be given choice-making opportunities and be rewarded for making choices.

How do we plan to meet the goals?

1. Every quarter, review teacher journal entries to examine the progress James is making
2. Weekly or bimonthly discussion with staff regarding James' Life Course IEP
3. Outcome journal notes shared with staff and family at scheduled meeting times

Benchmarks/Activities:

- James identifies the city bus route through pictured and GPS maps via electronic devices.
- James will ride the city bus with educational support staff and with his parents.
- James will hand money to the bus driver and greet "hello," use "thank you," and use appropriate leave-taking comments when exiting the bus, e.g., "goodbye."
- James will begin to make choices from "Stop and Think" prompts by the educational staff, such as, "James what do you think is best? Tell me where to put your backpack, ticket stub? Or, which bus stop will we get off at?"

Note: James currently understands and follows verbal instructions and will begin to comprehend Stop and Think prompts.

---

journal notes with the team and family requesting input and makes adjustments to the plan as needed.

Addressing transition goals for James at a young age gives him a head start on transitioning from school, obtaining employment, and living independently. It also sends a clear message to his parents that his educational team has similar hopes and dreams for James, and efforts toward realizing those dreams are in concert with their wishes.

Consultative Coaching and Life Course Outcome Mapping

Having a high-quality consultative coach to support transition across the life span aligns with best practice for educating students with ASD. In their respective roles, consultative coaches could offer mini-trainings on the use of the life course IEP, and explain how to set up the outcome journal. Consultant coaches could also be instrumental in setting up the initial dialogue with parents regarding their aspirations for their child. This level of coaching would provide the teacher with added support about the LCOM process and a chance to dialogue about benefits or downsides. The most important aspect about life course transition planning is that it is dialogical and collaborative in nature, stimulating discussion about what the student will do in the future. Consequently, relevant instructional approaches, particularly those that focus on spontaneous communication, might be well matched with the aims of many parents.

An HQC-A consultative coach also needs to have the requisite knowledge base to share up-to-date information so educational staff have an enhanced understanding of the purpose for implementation and the potential for long-term transition planning. A coach might share information about evidence-based interventions that are a strong match for a student's needs (e.g., visually supportive cues). Using visuals as instructional supports is especially helpful when an individual with ASD does not accurately interpret naturally occurring dynamic visual cues (Hayes et al., 2010). McKay, Weiss, Dickson, and Ahearn (2014) found that visual supports along with prompting hierarchies were effective strategies for teaching vocational skills for individuals with severe ASD and/or significant ID. Likewise, Sabielny and Cannella-Malone (2014) found the effectiveness of prompting strategies increased the efficiency of skill acquisition, reduced the number of errors, and avoided prompt dependency by individuals with ASD. In particular, these authors found that using a most-to-least prompting hierarchy tended to be more efficient and resulted in fewer errors than a least-to-most technique.

A potential drawback is that a consultant coach may overwhelm instructors with too much information without a strategy for implementation and follow-along, especially as it relates to transition. To avoid this obstacle, the coach might familiarize the teacher with a honed list of key resources, including evidence-based briefs and research articles or their abstracts to support the use of suggested instructional approaches with a given student. A consultative coach who takes the time to identify appropriate instructional resources encourages instructors to consider alternative approaches, stimulating conversation and encouraging implementation with an eye on the future.

Intensive Coaching and Life Course Outcome Mapping

Depending on need, intensive coaching may be better suited when a student reaches the age of 16, and a formal transition plan is first put in place. In this case, the coach would help the teacher and team members understand the intent of the law ensuring that all the required elements are satisfied in the transition plan. Novice or inexperienced teachers would profit from more intensive coaching sessions in which the various roles and responsibilities of new personnel and noneducational agencies that will be involved in the student's transition from school to work are the focus, and understanding how to implement goals associated with the plan. The coach could also review all of the life course IEPs to frame a more actionable picture for the teacher and staff.

Intensive coaches would be instrumental in a relatively new derivative of supported employment, called "customized employment" (Gerhardt & Lainer, 2011). The main idea of customized employment is highly specialized and focused on person-centered planning, or "job carving" that emphasizes the needs, interests, and abilities of both the employer and the employee. Customized employment results in meeting the needs of both parties involved: employer and potential employee. Some of the elements to consider in a supported environment are job training, continual job coaching, job modifications, and employee supervision by employers (Hagner & Cooney, 2005).

If a coach does not have a thorough understanding of transitioning options and the complexities associated with transition planning, teachers, staff, and parents may be asked to entertain service delivery options that are unclear. Therefore, the coach imparts founda-

tional knowledge in order to convey in a clear and concise manner the steps needed to make the transition from formal schooling to postschool life successful. Although a life course outcome map and life course IEP provide an operating framework, a coach also recognizes the limits of his or her own expertise. Hence, agencies who vendor postschool services and provide family and staff consultation are essential participants in the transition planning process as stipulated on the life course outcome map. The coach along with the educational team and family advocate for student self-reliance and target prevocational and vocational skills, while the student is still in school, so important for students with ASD once they enter the job market.

Summary

The number of children diagnosed with ASD has increased dramatically in the last 20 years (Centers for Disease Control and Prevention, 2014), and now these individuals are entering adulthood with limited vocational placements and very little opportunity for employment. This chapter began with a review of studies that have shown improved quality of life and cognitive performance for adults with ASD who are provided with supported employment. However, despite the positive impact of adult employment, families are left with fragmented systems of care once their youth with ASD transition out of entitled children's service system from IDEA into adulthood. Educational researchers suspect that current models of school-based transition planning are inadequate given these poor outcomes. Additionally, there is a shortage of appropriate opportunities for independence, and concurrently a long wait time for adults with ASD to receive postschool services.

To offset these startling trends, a life course outcome mapping along with a life course IEP provides a prospective planning framework for parents, caregivers, and educators to start an important conversation about life after formal schooling as soon as the child enters school. Life course outcome mapping is a practical alternative for educators, coaches, and families to begin transition planning as early as possible in a child's school career, from earliest entry to school exit.

High-quality coaching delivered at three levels (peer-to-peer, consultative, and intensive) using a life course outcome map ensures, at the very least, that the conversation about transition planning takes center stage as the student progresses into and beyond high school. The life course IEP also concretizes transition goals for parents very early in a child's educational career to maximize every opportunity to realize the hopes and aspirations all parents have for their children. Although the life course outcome map provides a framework for transition planning throughout school, high-quality coaching makes these goals actionable and attainable.

End-of-Chapter Questions

1. Consider the impact that life course planning could potentially have for students with ASD and their families. Read one article from the reference section of this chapter and summarize key points of the article. Be prepared to share them with colleagues at your school site, classmates, or via online discussion boards.

2. Develop a life course outcome map on one of your students with ASD, or a student you have opportunity to observe. As far as possible include parents in the conversation. Make sure your life course IEP goals accent the hopes and dreams of parents, and transition to postschool steps are clearly evident.

3. As a peer-to-peer coach, how would you use the life course outcome map you developed? Make sure to describe to your team implementation strategies. Be sure to discuss the importance of outcome journaling and scheduled debriefing regarding progress toward meeting the life course goals and benchmarks/activities.

4. Identify key support personnel for students beginning the transition at age 16. Role-play an intensive coaching situation where you are working with a teacher and staff of high school students on the autism spectrum. Your role as intensive coach is to help teacher and staff comprehend the complexities involved with transitioning from the safety net of formal schooling to real-world demands. You may need to review the Stewart et al. (2001) as well as Taylor et al. (2012, 2014) articles in the reference section prior to acting out the role-play.

References

Billstedt, E., Gillberg, I., & Gillberg, C. (2005). Autism after adolescence: Population-based 13- to 22-year follow-up study of 120 individuals with autism diagnosed in childhood. *Journal of Autism and Developmental Disorders, 35*(3), 351–360.

Building the Legacy of IDEA. (2004). IDEA Regulations, Secondary Transition. [34 CFR 300.43 (a)] [20 U.S.C. 1401(34)].

Centers for Disease Control and Prevention. (2014). *Autism spectrum disorder: data and statistics.* Retrieved July 16, 2015, from http://www.cdc.gov/ncbddd/autism/data.html

Clark, H., Knab, J., & Kincaid, D. (2005). Person-centered planning. In M. Hersen, J. Rosqvist, A. Gross, R. Drabman, G. Sugai, & R. Horner (Eds.), *Encyclopedia of behavior modification and cognitive behavior therapy: Volume 1, Adult clinical applications* (pp. 429–431). Thousand Oaks, CA: Sage.

Friedman, N., Warfield, M., & Parish, S. (2013). Transition to adulthood for individuals with autism spectrum disorder: Current issues and future perspectives. *Neuropsychiatry, 3*(2), 181.

Garcia, S. (2015). *Teaching vocational gardening skills to an adolescent with severe autism* (Unpublished master's thesis). California State University Monterey Bay, Seaside, CA.

Garcia-Villamisar, D., Wehman, P., & Diaz Navarro, M. (2002). Changes in the quality of autistic people's life that work in supported and sheltered employment. A 5-year follow-up study. *Journal of Vocational Rehabilitation, 17*, 309–312.

Gerhardt, P., & Lainer, I. (2011). Addressing the needs of adolescents and adults with autism: A crisis on the horizon. *Journal of Contemporary Psychotherapy, 41*(1), 37–45.

Hagner, D., & Cooney, B. (2005). "I do that for everybody": Supervising employees with autism. *Focus on Autism and Other Developmental Disabilities, 20*(2), 91–97.

Hayes, G., Hirano, S., Marcu, G., Monibi, M., & Nguyen, D. (2010). Interactive visual supports for children with autism. *Personal and Ubiquitous Computing, 14*(7), 663–680.

Howlin, P., Goode, S., Hutton, J., & Rutter, M. (2004). Adult outcome for children with autism. *Journal of Child Psychology and Psychiatry, 45*(2), 212–229.

King, G. A., Baldwin, P. J., Currie, M., & Evans, J. (2005). Planning successful transitions from school to adult roles for youth with disabilities. *Children's Health Care. 34*(3),193–216.

McKay, J., Weiss, J., Dickson, C., & Ahearn, W. (2014). Comparison of prompting hierarchies on acquisition of leisure and vocational skills. *Behavior Analysis in Practice, 7*(2), 91–102.

Migliore, A., Butterworth, J., & Zalewska, A. (2014). Trends in vocational rehabilitation services and outcomes of youth with autism: 2006–2010. *Rehabilitation Counseling Bulletin, 57*(2), 80–89.

Sabielny, L., & Cannella-Malone, H. (2014). Comparison of prompting strategies on the acquisition of daily living skills. *Education and Training in Autism and Developmental Disabilities, 49*(1), 145–152.

Stewart, D., Freeman, M., Law, M., Healy, H., Burke-Gaffney, J., Forhan, M., . . . Guenther, S. (2010). Transition to adulthood for youth with disabilities: Evidence from the literature. In J. H. Stone & M. Blouin (Eds.), *International encyclopedia of rehabilitation.* Center for International Rehabilitation Research Information and Exchange (CIRRIE), The State University of New York at Buffalo.

Stewart, D., Law, M., Rosenbaum, P., & Williams, D. G. (2001). A qualitative study of the transition to adulthood for youth with physical disabilities. *Physical and Occupational Therapy in Pediatrics, 21*(4), 3–21.

Taylor, J., & Seltzer, M. (2010). Changes in the autism behavioral phenotype during the transition to adulthood. *Journal of Autism and Developmental Disorders, 40*(12), 1431–1446.

Taylor, J., & Seltzer, M. (2012). Developing a vocational index for adults with autism spectrum disorders. *Journal of Autism and Developmental Disorders, 42*(12), 2669–2679.

Taylor, J., Smith, L., & Mailick, M. (2014). Engagement in vocational activities pro-motes behavioral development for adults with autism spectrum disorders. *Journal of Autism and Developmental Disorders, 44*(6), 1447–1460.

Turnbull, A. (2010). *Transitioning to enviable lives for adults with autism.* Geneva Centre International Symposium on Autism. Retrieved July 16, 2015, from http://www.cmcgc.com/media/handouts/101103/140_Ann_Turnbull.pdf

Wehman, P. (2013). *Life beyond the classroom: Transition strategies for young people with disabilities* (5th ed.). Baltimore, MD: Paul H. Brookes.

CHAPTER 13

Embedding High-Quality Coaching at the District Level: Establishing a Network of Coaches

Leadership and learning are indispensable to each other.
—John F. Kennedy

Chapter Objectives

- Understand the importance of building local capacity for coaching as a means of serving students with autism spectrum disorder (ASD).

- Note obstacles to local capacity building.

- Recruit teams and build coaching networks.

Introduction

Administrators and staff in public school districts understand that the rising prevalence of students with ASD necessitates services that are as comprehensive as possible so that these students can remain in their neighborhood schools. How do school districts begin the process of implementing high-quality coaching that aligns with evidence-based assessment and instructional practices in serving students with ASD? A recommended approach is to install a service delivery model that builds district capacity to serve students locally, rather than relying on agencies hired from the outside to do this for them. While contracting with outside agencies can be a great way to introduce the systematic utilization of evidence-based interventions (EBIs) in autism programs across the district, there are some disadvantages to long-term reliance on them. For example, programming costs can spiral upward and, at the same time, decisions about methodology may be ceded to the instructional philosophy of the contracting agency. Whereas local school districts need to focus on providing programming sufficiently broad in scope to address the range of core challenges seen among students with ASD as well as the preferences of families (National Research Council, 2001), independent agencies are more likely to deliver interventions that are narrow in focus and that align with their foundational pedagogy. Even though a specific intervention process like the vignette described with Mrs. Tracy in Chapter 8

(see Box 8–1) may appeal to some families, agency personnel trained to deliver a methodology consistent with a single instructional philosophy delimits programming options for a school district. For example, a discrete trial teaching approach may take precedence over curricular and teaching approaches in the classroom necessitating instructional and supervisorial staff from the agency that can overwhelm the ratio of adults to students and co-opt teacher control. We previously addressed this obstacle in Section 1 (see Chapter 1) with the "Buyer's Remorse" vignette when too many adults changed the dynamics of the classroom (see Box 1–5). Consequently, a strong motivation for many school districts in building their own coaching networks is to retain pedagogical control. Experts in the field of ASD have forcefully endorsed the recommendation for training teachers with a variety of evidence-based approaches in ASD classrooms to avoid "rigidity in training" (see coaching obstacles in Chapter 1). Rigidity in training can impact the continuity of programming as students move to other programs or schools within a school district, as well as precipitate unnecessary legal challenges by parents brought against local school districts (Scheuermann et al., 2003).

The decision about whether to bring in outside consulting agencies depends on district priorities and programmatic needs. For example, teachers may require assistance with deepening their skills to implement specific EBIs in the classroom. Alternatively, a district or school site may need professional development training for general education staff lacking background knowledge about ASD and the range of characteristics associated with students with this disability. Whatever the goal, it is wise to establish clear outcomes and goals to be evaluated at end of a consultative arrangement to determine next steps. Contracts that are time-limited are typically advisable over those that extend from one academic year to the next. Even public educational agencies tasked to provide this kind of resource at no expense to local districts need to fade involvement over time, so that local teaching staff can achieve a level of independence and confidence in providing for students with ASD.

Forming a District Autism Leadership Team

In this book, we have built the argument that educators in public settings can build internal capacity and competent delivery through the provision of a tiered coaching system. As emphasized previously in Section 1, coaching support begins with an inviting partner and typically an expert in evidence-based strategies for students with ASD, or a specialist recruited to address the needs of a particular student, teacher, or program. However, to ensure that these effective coaching practices are fully embedded across all classrooms for children with ASD in a school district, strong leadership and systematic support at the district level will be critical.

To achieve this outcome, it is imperative that a group of individuals, tasked with the development, implementation, and monitoring of autism programs within schools and/or across the district be established. An "Autism Leadership Team" would oversee the implementation of effective, multilevel coaching practices to support educators of students with ASD in the district. As such, careful consideration should be made to identify potential members of this team. Given that the purview of the team will be district programming for the unique needs of individuals with ASD, it will be essential to recruit the leadership of the district special education director (or, administrative designee in very large districts). If the district provides regional or grade-level assistant directors, these individuals would be ideal team members as well. Individuals responsible for arranging professional development in the area of ASD should also participate. Districts should consider recruiting parents or family members of students with ASD to collaborate on the leadership team. Last, if the district is contracting with outside experts or agencies, these individuals (or representatives) should be invited to participate with the team, as again the goal of involving outside expertise is ultimately to build the district's own capacity.

The autism leadership team as it evolves should meet on a monthly (or at least quarterly) basis, and follow the effective meeting recommendations covered in Chapter 6, such as identifying team member roles, using an agenda, developing and following action plans, and so on. As a district leadership team on ASD, activities of the team will be focused on enhancing the capabilities of the district to implement and sustain effective, multilevel coaching supports to teachers in providing effective, evidence-based interventions for students. The autism leadership team could further engage in defining clear objectives, such as allocating resources to support coaching practices, building networks of coaches, working with outside experts and agencies to enhance district capacity to implement effective programming for students with ASD, and evaluate, develop, and recommend district policies to this end. Additional considerations for each of these important objectives are discussed in the following sections.

Allocating Coaching Resources

As described in previous chapters, teachers may need higher-intensity coaching in all areas of instruction (all chapters in Section II), or they may only require higher-intensity coaching in a few (or even just one) specific areas. Therefore, a central focus of the autism leadership team will be to ensure that an adequate number of individuals is made available to coach teachers with varying levels of need. A first step toward this goal would be to review, or if necessary conduct, a staff inventory (names, assignments, credentials held, areas of strength/need, etc.) to identify the potential areas and

levels of coaching support needed by educators across the district. District coaches could then be matched to educators based on this information. This would also allow the leadership team to identify if adequate coaching supports currently exist in the district, or if action planning on building these supports will need to be conducted by the leadership team. One potentially critical activity in ensuring that adequate coaching supports are available involves the funding of personnel to conduct coaching activities. The leadership team will likely need to develop action plan activities to determine the best ways to allocate full-time equivalence (FTE) to personnel involved in supporting teachers with coaching activities, particularly at the consultative and intensive coaching levels. Likewise, the team may need to think creatively about maximizing their efficiency in using personnel to implement coaching. For example, some districts may choose to embed coaching responsibilities by existing professionals already tasked to provide mentorship supports to teachers. Mentor teachers, while perhaps not sufficiently available to provide intensive coaching, may nonetheless be ideally suited to implement consultative and peer-to-peer coaching strategies. Furthermore, ensuring that the responsibilities expected of those in the coaching role are written into job descriptions and position announcements is a critical step toward impacting the long-term sustainability of effective coaching supports.

Additionally, given the need for coaches to possess a level of expertise in effective services for students with ASD and in effective coaching approaches, the leadership team may want to arrange for and provide professional development activities that directly address coaches' needs in the district. Surveying coaches to identify areas of professional development in supporting the teachers they work with is an effective way to discover and prioritize these activities.

Building Coaching Networks

As previously discussed, in order to support all who provide for the needs of children with ASD across an educational agency, a number of individuals will likely play the role of coach in all but the smallest of districts. Therefore, it will be advantageous for districts to not only invest in providing resources to coaches, as described in the previous section, but to also invest in the sustainability of coaching practices across the district. One way to achieve this is through the establishment of a coaching network. With a coaching network, an autism leadership team might convene periodic meetings of all district coaches (or just coaches providing consultative or intensive coaching) to engage in structured discussions about coaching experiences and strategies, issues with assembling and working with educational teams (i.e., content in Chapter 6), conducting meaningful assessments to inform instruction (i.e., content in Chapters 7 and 8), and problem solving particular implementation issues with various

EBIs (i.e., content in Chapters 9, 10, and 11), and so on. The contact information of members of the coaching network should be shared among coaches allowing for ongoing collaboration, problem solving, and moral support. Additionally, a portion of the district website could be made available just for members of the leadership team and coaching network. This could function as a local clearinghouse for coaches including resources from other professional development activities or professional organizations (e.g., OCALI Autism Internet Modules, cited in Chapter 9, Box 9–1). The website could also be used to periodically post discussion board topics submitted by coaches and to generate responses from others.

Working With Outside Experts to Build Capacity

Another important role of the autism leadership team is to evaluate the need for, and oversee the services provided by outside experts and/or agencies providing autism-related services in the district. As previously articulated, the role of the outside expert/agency should be that of district capacity builder, and not simply that of "hired hand." As such, the leadership team will need to be clear in the contractual process regarding expectations as to how agency expert(s) will enhance the district's ability to operate independently in the service areas being provided.

Upon entering into such a relationship, the leadership team should establish specific required qualifications held by the expert/agency. Fortunately, a growing number of organizations have established common certification requirements and professional and ethical guidelines for the professionals to whom they grant certification. For example, the Behavior Analyst Certification Board® has established very clear qualification criteria for the various levels of certification it provides, along with a comprehensive Professional and Ethical Compliance Code for Behavior Analysts (Behavior Analyst Certification Board®, 2014). Members of the autism leadership team would do well to familiarize themselves with the qualification criteria of various credential, certification, and endorsement agencies, along with the professional and ethical guidelines set by the organizations that oversee the ongoing conduct of their members.

When entering into a consultative relationship with an outside expert/agency, the leadership team should also establish clear project outcomes and goals to be evaluated over time to guide the focus of external supports to be provided. At the end of the contractual period, these outcomes and goals should be evaluated in order to make informed decisions about the need or desire for continued services from the specialist or contracting agency. An example would be where a district team identifies a comprehensive evidence-based intervention (EBI) to be added to the repertoire of a number of teachers and coaches in the district. Members of the district team draft a summary of activities to be performed by the external service provider, including direct service provision, and also activities to build the skills of educators and coaches to independently implement the practice. The summary of outcomes and objectives should also outline the qualifications of the outside consultant/group, the expectations for the shadowing of the expert(s)/agency personnel in district classrooms and with district personnel, and the gradual release of modeling and consultative activities to district personnel. The expert or agency would be expected to participate with the autism leadership team meetings by reporting progress made on all of these activities. In this example, the leadership team would also want to have knowledge of and influence on the budget available for these services. With these pieces of information, bids from experts/agencies could be solicited by the school district, with as much involvement of the leadership team as possible in the selection of an appropriate expert/agency.

Influencing District Policy

Given its leadership function, it is appropriate for an autism leadership team to draft and otherwise seek to influence the development of district policies designed to ensure and promote the effectiveness of programming across the district for individuals with ASD. One area in which teams may want to focus is the development of district policies regarding the importance of only using EBIs. Also, teams may want to develop district policy on the issue of contracting with outside experts and agencies, to clarify the need for these external services in serving a capacity-building role for the district. Additional areas of focus for policy development could include guidelines on position descriptions related to coaching, teacher evaluation procedures, full-time equivalent (FTE) allocations for coaching responsibilities, and so on.

Summary

When seeking to embed effective coaching practices to support teachers working with students with ASD within the school district, numerous system-level reforms at the district level may be warranted. A district autism leadership team can assume the burden of initiating, implementing, and evaluating these efforts. Ultimately, to build the district's own capacity to implement EBIs with students with ASD, district leaders will need to enhance their own knowledge and skills in these areas. Further, the district will need to provide leadership and support to the individuals providing coaching to teachers in effective instruction. To affect systems change in programming for individuals with ASD, the district leadership team must consist of members with decision-making authority as well as a commitment to support the development of strong coach and teacher relationships.

End-of-Chapter Questions

1. Write a sample district policy on the use of evidence-based interventions for students with ASD.

2. Develop a sample agenda for an ASD Coaching Network meeting. What conversation starters would you select? What activities would you identify? What would be the objectives of the meeting?

3. Your district is planning to extend a contract to an outside consulting agency to initiate the implementation of an evidence-based intervention for students with ASD. What attributes would you want this agency to possess and why?

References

Behavior Analyst Certification Board®. (2014). *Professional and ethical compliance code for behavior analysts.* Littleton, CO: Behavior Analyst Certification Board®.

National Research Council. (2001). *Educating children with autism.* Washington, DC: National Academy of Sciences, National Academy Press.

Scheuermann, B., Webber, J., Boutot, E. A., & Goodwin, M. (2003). Problems with personnel preparation in autism spectrum disorders. *Focus on Autism and Other Developmental Disabilities, 18,* 197–206.

Index

Note: Page numbers in **bold** reference non-text material.

Trainers, expert, 70
Training
  Behavior Skills Training (BST), 45–46, **46**
  rigidity in, 230
Training teachers, 40, **40**
Transition planning, 209–228
  initial planning at school entry, 214–220
  Life Course Outcome Mapping, 213–220, **222–223**, 224–226
  Life Course Outcome Mapping form, **218–219**
  nontraditional, 213–214
  traditional, 213
  vignettes, **210**, **215**
Transition services, 210–211
Treatment and Research Institute for ASDs (TRIAD), Vanderbilt University, **124**
Trials to criterion data collection
  example form, **144**
  methods, 142–144

U

University of California, Davis, **150**
University of California, Santa Barbara, 203

V

VBIE coaching. *See* Virtual bug-in-the-ear coaching
Video modeling
  combined with peer-mediated instruction, **167**, 167–170, **168–169**
  for social communication skills, 166
Video self-modeling, 154–157
Virtual bug-in-the-ear (VBIE) coaching, 46–48, **47**
Virtual delivery methods, 46–48
Visual supports, 224
VM. *See* Video modeling
Vocational rehabilitation, 212

W

Weekly schedules, 81–82
Work samples, **121**
Written text cues, 166

Y

Yale *in Vivo* Pragmatic Protocol, **124**